Anatomy Tutor for Surgeons in Training

A multiple-choice tutor in anatomy

Anatomy Tutor for Surgeons in Training
A multiple-choice tutor in anatomy

Reuben D. Johnson BSc, MBChB (Glas)

Arun Sahai BSc, MBBS (Lond)
Jonothan Epstein MA (Cantab), BMBCh (Oxon)
Anant Krishnan BSc, MBBS (Lond)
Alexis Schizas BSc, MBBS (Lond)
Paul Patterson MBBS (Lond), FRCS (Edin)

Foreword by Professor Harold Ellis CBE, FRCS

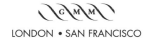

LONDON • SAN FRANCISCO

GMM

www.greenwich-medical.co.uk

© 2003
Greenwich Medical Media Limited
137 Euston Road
London
NW1 2AA

870 Market Street, Ste 720
San Francisco
CA 94102

ISBN 1841101362

First Published 2003

Design by Bright Yellow Design & Marketing

Typeset by Mizpah Publishing Services, Chennai, India

Printed in the UK by the Alden Group, Oxford

Distributed by Plymbridge Distributors Ltd and in the USA by Jamco Distribution

CONTENTS

FOREWORD

The multiple-choice question (MCQ) is now an established part of the examination system in the UK and in many other countries. Of course, it has its disadvantages – it is impersonal, it does not test the candidate's ability to express himself or herself in English or to display the process of logical thought (but other parts of most examination systems do this), and it lacks fine gradations of meaning. Yet it does enable a wide range of factual knowledge to be tested in a relatively short time, and no-one can accuse the computer of being biased, racist or sexist, or of marking unfairly! It also serves another useful purpose, in that books of MCQs such as this check the knowledge store and ensure that at least the essentials of any programme of study have been absorbed.

I have had the enjoyable experience of working my way through this volume, written by a keen team of young surgeons, all but one of whom are still in training. If it is of any satisfaction to the reader, I confess that I made some mistakes, although none that I would have considered life-threatening to my patients. There are, of course, no substitutes for practical work in the dissecting room, the study of the disarticulated skeleton, the perusal of a good textbook and, perhaps best of all, expertise in living surface anatomy. However, by carefully working through this book, and checking up any errors or gaps in your knowledge that crop up, you will have a valuable revision, as well as an excellent preparation for your MCQ examination in anatomy.

Harold Ellis CBE, FRCS
January 2002

PREFACE

This concise book has been compiled by a group of doctors who, with the single exception of Paul Patterson, were Anatomy Demonstrators at Guy's, King's and St Thomas's (GKT) School of Medicine and Biomedical Sciences, where they studied anatomy under Professor Harold Ellis in preparation for postgraduate surgical examinations. They are now surgical trainees, having completed posts in Accident and Emergency at either King's College or St Thomas's Hospital. Paul Patterson graduated from University College London, and has worked in London, Newcastle and Glasgow; he is now a Registrar in Orthopaedics in Boston, Lincolnshire.

The book is based primarily on the authors' tutorials and dissection sessions held at Guy's Campus for the preclinical medical and dental courses; clinically oriented questions on limb and joint anatomy have been compiled by Paul Patterson.

Each chapter begins with a topic list designed to help the student plan and coordinate a programme of study. MCQs have been designed to illustrate the main points of each topic and are accompanied by full text answers to help students acquire and consolidate their knowledge of anatomy. Diagrams have been included which the authors have found useful, both in teaching students at GKT and in passing their own surgical examinations.

The text will prove invaluable for both medical and dental students, and for those intending to sit, and pass, the MCQ component of the Member of the Royal College of Surgeons (MRCS) examination.

In writing this volume, we are indebted to our teachers, and in particular to Professor Harold Ellis and the late Mr Roger Parker, who have inspired us through their own teaching and their enthusiasm for clinical anatomy. We would also like to express our gratitude to Mr A.T. Raftery, Consultant Surgeon with the Sheffield Teaching Hospitals NHS Trust and examiner for the Royal College of Surgeons of England, for his kindness in reading through our manuscript with such diligence and for his advice and encouragement. We are grateful to Mr Geoff Nuttall and Mr Gavin Smith of Greenwich Medical Media for publishing this volume.

Reuben D. Johnson
January 2002

AUTHORS

Reuben D. Johnson, BSc (Hons), MBChB (Glas)
Demonstrator in Anatomy
Guy's, King's and St Thomas's
SHO in Accident and Emergency
King's College Hospital, London

Arun Sahai, BSc (Hons), MBBS (Lond)
Demonstrator in Anatomy
Guy's, King's and St Thomas's
SHO in Accident and Emergency
St Thomas's Hospital, London

Jonothan Epstein, MA (Cantab), BMBCh (Oxon)
Demonstrator in Anatomy
Guy's, King's and St Thomas's
SHO in Accident and Emergency
King's College Hospital, London

Anant Krishnan, BSc (Hons), MBBS (Lond)
Demonstrator in Anatomy
Guy's, King's and St Thomas's
SHO in Accident and Emergency
St Thomas's Hospital, London

Alexis Schizas, BSc (Hons), MBBS (Lond)
Demonstrator in Anatomy
Guy's, King's and St Thomas's
SHO in Accident and Emergency
King's College Hospital, London

Paul Patterson, MBBS (Lond), FRCS (Edin)
Specialist Registrar in Orthopaedics
Boston, Lincolnshire

INTRODUCTION

This volume has been written with both MRCS candidates and undergraduate students of anatomy in mind. As most preclinical medical courses and postgraduate medical examinations contain MCQs, it has become advantageous for students to practise large numbers of this type of question, so as to familiarise themselves with the technique. Unfortunately, this is often at the expense of mastering the subject matter by reading a comprehensive text. We have endeavoured to help candidates overcome this problem by writing longer and more in-depth answers to questions than is usual in the great majority of MCQ books. Each answer summarises the main points of anatomy which must be grasped in order to answer the question, and includes helpful tips for remembering these points.

The book has been divided into chapters which reflect the areas of the human body dissected and taught separately in most medical schools. Each chapter begins with a check list: this structures the information relating to the anatomical area by dividing it into a series of themes which, in their turn, give rise to more specific topics; each topic corresponds to a numbered question. In this way, the reader can see clearly the essential points of anatomy with which it is necessary to become familiar. This will also facilitate the acquisition of anatomical knowledge in the dissection room and in private reading.

We have included diagrams that we have found useful in teaching students at Guy's, King's and St Thomas's School of Medicine. These diagrams are intended to help clarify, or to summarise, the information given in the text. Students may find it useful to re-draw these diagrams themselves and to commit them to memory.

Reuben D. Johnson
January 2002

1. Thorax

TOPIC CHECK LIST

THORACIC CAGE AND CONTENTS

1. Regions of the thorax.

A. The thymus gland is usually found in the anterior mediastinum.

B. The mediastinum is separated into superior and inferior by a line drawn horizontally backwards from the 3rd costal cartilage.

C. In the posterior mediastinum the thoracic duct lies posterior to the oesophagus.

D. In the superior mediastinum the brachiocephalic veins unite to form the superior vena cava (SVC) at the level of T4/T5.

E. The branches of the arch of the aorta lie anterior to the brachiocephalic veins, in the superior mediastinum.

True:	C D
False:	A B E

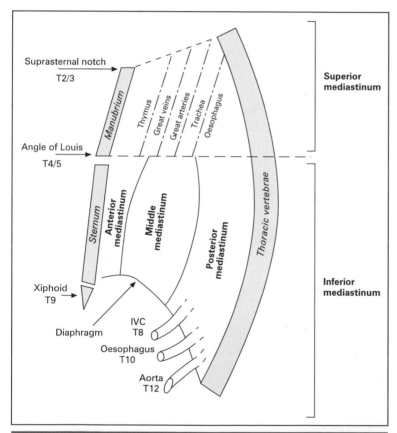

Fig. 1 Lateral view of the thorax, showing the division of the mediastinum into superior and inferior regions. The inferior mediastinum is further subdivided into anterior, middle and posterior regions. Note the relations of structures in the superior mediastinum, and also the levels at which the inferior vena cava (IVC), oesophagus and aorta pass through the diaphragm in the abdomen.

The mediastinum, the space in between the pleura, is separated into superior and inferior by a line drawn horizontally from the sternal angle, at the level of T4/T5. The inferior mediastinum is further subdivided into anterior, middle and posterior. The superior mediastinum, from anterior to posterior, contains the thymus gland, brachiocephalic veins, branches of the arch of the aorta, the trachea, oesophagus, thoracic duct, thoracic sympathetic chain and finally the vertebral column. In addition, it also harbours the vagi, phrenic and left recurrent laryngeal nerves. In the posterior mediastinum, the thoracic duct, azygos vein, thoracic vertebrae and descending thoracic aorta (near the diaphragm) are all posterior relations of the oesophagus. The anterior mediastinum essentially contains some lymph nodes and the internal thoracic vessels. The middle mediastinum contents include the heart and great vessels. *See Figure 1.*

2.   The surface anatomy of the thorax.

A.   The angle of Louis (sternal angle) lies at the level of T4/T5.

B.   The right pleural edge crosses the 10th rib in the mid-clavicular line (MCL).

C.   The medial border of the scapula can approximate the oblique fissure of the lungs when the shoulder is fully abducted.

D.   The lowest part of the costal margin corresponds to the 10th rib, which lies at the level of L2.

E.   The pleura descend below the 12th rib at its medial extremity.

True:	A C E
False:	B D

The pleura extend approximately 1 in. (2.5 cm) above the clavicle and descend below the 12th rib margin at its medial extremity. Ribs 6, 8, 10 (lungs) and 8, 10, 12 (pleura) refer to the lower limits of the lungs and pleura as they cross the MCL, the mid-axillary line (MAL) and the lateral border of erector spinae, respectively. The oblique fissure, which divides the lungs into upper and lower lobes, can be represented by fully abducting the shoulder. The line of the oblique fissure corresponds to the medial border of the scapula. The transverse fissure separates the middle and upper lobes of the right lung. Its surface marking is a line drawn horizontally along the 4th costal cartilage, meeting the oblique fissure as it crosses the 5th rib.

Some important surface anatomy in the thorax:

- Suprasternal notch (T2)
- Angle of Louis (T4/T5)
- Xiphisternum (T9)
- Lowest part of costal margin (10th rib, L3)

3.   The ribs.

A.   Ribs 8 and 9 are typical ribs.

B.   The tubercle of a typical rib articulates with the transverse process of the vertebral body above.

C.   The head of a typical rib articulates with a thoracic intervertebral disc.

D.   The head of a typical rib has a single facet which articulates with the corresponding vertebral body.

E.   The term 'false' rib refers to the floating ribs 11 and 12 alone.

True:	A C
False:	B D E

Ribs are classified into typical and atypical, true and false ribs. It is essential to have a thorough understanding of these terms. Typical ribs have a head, neck, tubercle, angle and shaft. The head has two demi-facets (upper and lower) separated by a crest. The lower demi-facet articulates with the corresponding vertebral body (e.g., 3rd rib with T3) and the upper demi-facet with the vertebral body above (e.g., 3rd rib with T2). The crest, therefore, articulates with the intervening IV disc (e.g., 3rd rib with the IV disc between T2 and T3). The tubercle of a typical rib has a facet which articulates with the transverse process of the corresponding vertebra (e.g., 3rd rib with T3). The shaft, or body, of a typical rib is flat in the vertical plane and has a groove on its inner lower surface for the passage of the intercostal neurovascular (NV) bundle. The features of a typical rib are shown in *Figure 2*. Any rib that does not conform to this pattern is an atypical rib. The first rib is atypical because it is flat in a horizontal plane, it has a single facet on its head, and its tubercle is on its inner border (known as the scalene tubercle). Ribs 10, 11 and 12 are atypical because they have only a single facet on their heads, by which they articulate with the bodies of their corresponding vertebrae. In addition, ribs 11 and 12 have no tubercles.

The distinction between a true rib and false rib lies in whether or not the costal cartilages at the front of the ribs articulate directly with the sternum. The cartilages of ribs 1–7 all articulate directly with the sternum and are therefore true ribs. The remaining five ribs are all false ribs. The 8th, 9th and 10th costal cartilages connect to the sternum indirectly by articulating with the 7th costal cartilage. The 11th and 12th costal cartilages have no attachment to the sternum and are also known as floating ribs.

Note: *See* the chapter on 'the vertebral column' for an account of a typical thoracic vertebra.

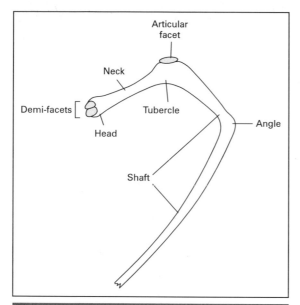

Fig. 2 Features of a typical rib.

---

4. The 1st rib.

A.   The 1st rib attaches the scalenus anterior muscle to its scalene tubercle.

B.   The 1st rib attaches serratus anterior superiorly.

C.   The subclavian artery and the root of the 1st thoracic spinal nerve cross posterior to the scalene tubercle.

D.   The subclavian vein crosses anterior to the scalene tubercle.

E.   The head of the 1st rib articulates with the body of C7 and T1.

True:	A B C D
False:	E

The 1st rib is flattened in the horizontal plane and is the shortest and most curved of all the ribs. Its head has a single facet which articulates with the body of T1. An important landmark is the scalene tubercle, which is found on its inner aspect for the attachment of scalenus anterior. Scalenus medius attaches posteriorly. The subclavian artery and root of T1 cross the body of the rib between scalenus anterior and medius, whereas the subclavian vein crosses anterior to the scalene tubercle. The 1st digit of serratus anterior attaches to the superior aspect of the 1st rib. The attachments and relations of the 1st rib are shown in *Figure 3*.

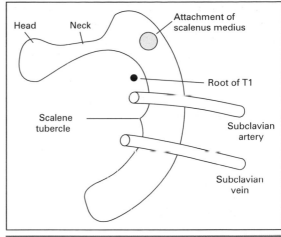

Fig. 3 The 1st rib and superior relations.

A.   The NV bundle lies between the external and internal intercostal muscles.

B.   The posterior intercostal arteries are all derived from the thoracic aorta.

C.   The anterior intercostal arteries supply the breast.

D.   The intercostal nerves supply the thoracic and abdominal walls.

E.   It is safe to insert a needle into the intercostal space, immediately below a rib.

| **True:** | **C D** |

| **False:** | **A B E** |

The intercostal space comprises (from the outside in) the external intercostal, internal intercostal and innermost intercostal muscles. The innermost is incompletely separated from the internal intercostal by the NV bundle. It is important to remember that the NV bundle lies below the rib: from above downwards, vein, artery, nerve (VAN). Thus, if one were to insert a needle into the chest for the purpose of aspiration, or a chest tube for drainage, one would aim superior to a rib to avoid hitting the NV bundle and possible subsequent haemorrhage. The intercostal nerves not only supply the muscles in the space but also give off cutaneous branches, which

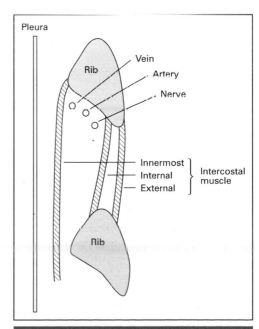

Fig. 4 The intercostal space in cross-section, showing the location and relations of the intercostal vein, artery and nerve.

supply the thoracic and abdominal walls. The subclavian artery, *via* its costocervical trunk, provides blood supply to the posterior 1st and 2nd spaces, whilst the rest of the posterior intercostal arteries are derived from the descending thoracic aorta. Anteriorly, the intercostal arteries are derived from the internal thoracic artery, another branch of the subclavian. This artery can be found one finger's-breadth away from the sternum, running down the chest wall. In the female, the branches of the anterior intercostal arteries, in the 2nd–4th spaces, are large and supply the breast. There is a rich anastomosis between the anterior and posterior intercostal arteries.

Note: A commonly asked question by examiners is to discuss the layers traversed by inserting either a needle in the 2nd intercostal space, MCL, or a tube in the 5th intercostal space, MAL. *Figure 4* illustrates the intercostal space.

6.	**Muscular attachments to the outer surface of the thoracic cage.**

A. The external oblique muscle (EOM) of the abdominal wall attaches to the lower four ribs only.

B. Serratus anterior attaches to the upper eight ribs.

C. Pectoralis major is supplied by the supraclavicular nerves from the cervical plexus.

D. Latissimus dorsi attaches to the lower four ribs and is supplied by the intercostal nerves 6, 7 and 8.

E. Rectus sternalis, the thoracic continuation of the rectus abdominis muscle (RAM), is present only in dogs.

True:	**B**
False:	**A C D E**

There are five muscles attaching to the shafts of the ribs and the costal cartilages: pectoralis major; pectoralis minor; serratus anterior; external oblique; and latissimus dorsi. Pectoralis major has two heads: a clavicular head from the medial two-thirds of the clavicle and the manubrium, and a sternocostal head from the 2nd to the 5th ribs and costal cartilages. Pectoralis major extends to the outer lip of the bicipital groove of the humerus. Pectoralis minor attaches the 3rd, 4th and 5th ribs and extends to the coracoid process of the scapula (considered in more detail in the chapter on 'upper limb'). While serratus anterior attaches to the outer aspects of the shafts of the upper eight ribs, the EOM of the anterior abdominal wall has attachments to the outer aspect of the shafts of the lower eight ribs. Latissimus dorsi attaches to the outer aspect of the

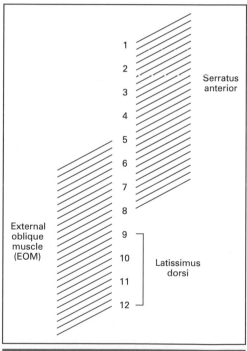

Fig. 5 Diagram summarising how the serratus anterior, external oblique muscle (EOM) and latissimus dorsi attach to the outer surface of the ribs. The finger-like fibres of serratus anterior attach to the upper eight ribs. These fibres interdigitate with EOM, which attaches to the lower eight ribs; latissimus dorsi attaches to the lower four ribs.

lower four ribs and extends to the bicipital groove of the humerus where it lies between the attachments of pectoralis major and teres major (a situation easily remembered by the mnemonic 'the lady in bed between the two majors'). *Figure 5* shows the attachments of the serratus anterior, latissimus dorsi and EOM. The thoracic attachments and nerve supply of these muscles are summarised below.

- Pectoralis major and minor: medial and lateral pectoral nerves (brachial plexus).
- Serratus anterior: long thoracic nerve (C5, 6, 7 brachial plexus).
- Latissimus dorsi: thoracodorsal nerve (C6, 7 and 8 brachial plexus).
- EOM: lower six thoracic nerves, iliohypogastric and ilioinguinal nerves (L1).

The rectus sternalis muscle is always present in dogs and was mistakenly described by Galen as being a constant muscle of human anatomy. It was the great Andreas Vesalius who pointed out that, although a vestigial rectus sternalis *may* occur in man, it is absent in most people.

7. Blood supply of the thoracic cage.

A. There are no vessels running along the top of a rib.

B. The hemiazygos system drains the left side of the chest wall into the inferior vena cava (IVC).

C. All the posterior intercostal arteries are derived from the descending thoracic aorta.

D. The anterior intercostal arteries arise from the internal thoracic (internal mammary) artery.

E. The internal thoracic arteries terminate as the single superior epigastric artery.

True:	D
False:	A B C E

The small collateral branches of the intercostal vessels run along the top of the ribs. The 1st and 2nd posterior intercostal arteries are derived from the costocervical trunk of the subclavian artery, but the rest are direct branches of the descending thoracic aorta. The posterior intercostal arteries form anastomoses with the anterior intercostals which are branches of the internal thoracic artery in the MCL. This artery finishes by dividing into the musculophrenic artery and the superior epigastric artery. This latter artery forms an important anastomosis with the inferior epigastric artery in the rectus sheath of the anterior abdominal wall (*see* chapter on 'abdomen'). The hemiazygos system is a highly variable system of veins, which drain the left side of the chest wall. Blood from the hemiazygos system crosses the mid-line to drain into the azygos system, which then drains into the SVC. Thus, all the blood from the whole thoracic cage drains into the SVC.

RESPIRATORY APPARATUS

8. The trachea.

A. The trachea is approximately 6 in. (15 cm) long.

B. The carina is at the level of the angle of Louis (T4/T5).

C. The isthmus of the thyroid crosses the 4th tracheal cartilage.

D. The trachea begins at the level of C5.

E. The trachea is a palpable structure in the living subject.

True:	B E
False:	A C D

The trachea (see Figure 6) begins at the level of C6, continuing 4.3 in. (11 cm) inferiorly from the cricoid cartilage to its bifurcation (the carina) at the level of the angle of Louis (T4/T5). It has a number of U-shaped cartilaginous rings and the isthmus of the thyroid crosses the 2nd ring in the neck. The trachea is an important surface landmark in the living subject and should be palpated routinely in examination of patients. A trachea that is deviated from the mid-line may indicate the presence of a tension pneumothorax on the opposite side of the chest (see later).

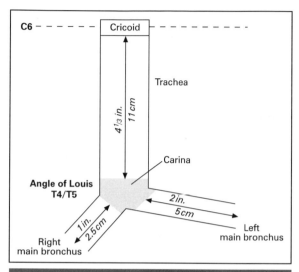

Fig. 6 The trachea and main bronchi. Note that the right main bronchus is shorter, wider and more vertical than the left: this explains why inhaled foreign bodies most commonly enter the right main bronchus.

9. The bronchial tree.

A. An inhaled foreign body most commonly travels down the left main bronchus.

B. The right main bronchus is longer than the left main bronchus.

C. The right main bronchus is crossed by the arch of the aorta.

D. The left main bronchus gives off three lobar bronchi.

E. A bronchopulmonary segment consists of branches of the pulmonary and bronchial vessels around a lobar bronchus.

All false.

The right main bronchus is shorter (1 in., or 2.5 cm), wider, and more vertical than the left main bronchus (2 in., or 5 cm) and is therefore the route taken most commonly by inhaled foreign bodies. The aorta arches to the left and the right main bronchus is crossed by the azygos vein which drains into the SVC. The main bronchi branch into lobar bronchi, which in turn branch into the tertiary bronchi. The left lung, having only two lobes, has two lobar bronchi. However, the lingular bronchus is sometimes considered to be a 'third lobar bronchus' although it is a branch of the upper lobar bronchus rather than the left main bronchus. The tertiary bronchi form the basis of a bronchopulmonary segment. These wedge-shaped functional units can be individually resected surgically.

10. The lungs.

A. The lingula of the right lung is equivalent to the third lobe.

B. The surface marking of the oblique fissure approximates to the 5th intercostal space.

C. The transverse fissure of the right lung approximates to the 6th costal cartilage.

D. The apex of the lung can be damaged by a knife wound above the clavicle.

E. A shallow stab wound at the level of the 9th rib in the mid-clavicular line may puncture the lung.

True:	B D
False:	**A C E**

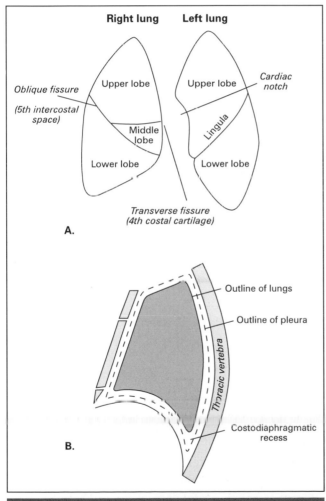

A.

Right lung Left lung

Oblique fissure
(5th intercostal space)

Upper lobe

Upper lobe

Cardiac notch

Middle lobe

Lingula

Lower lobe

Lower lobe

Transverse fissure
(4th costal cartilage)

B.

Outline of lungs

Outline of pleura

Thoracic vertebra

Costodiaphragmatic recess

Fig. 7 A. Lungs seen from the front, showing lobes and fissures.
B. A sagittal section of the thorax, showing outlines of lungs and pleura, and the costodiaphragmatic recess inferiorly (a potential space).

Figure 7 shows the lungs from the front, and also presents a sagittal section of the thorax, showing the pleura and lungs. The right lung has three lobes divided by the oblique and transverse fissures. The oblique fissure approximates to the 5th intercostal space at the surface of the lung. The transverse fissure approximates to a horizontal line from the 4th costal cartilage anteriorly. The left lung has two proper lobes and the lingula; the lingula can be considered to be the third lobe, which has regressed to make room for the heart. Due to the oblique slope of the 1st rib, the lung extends above the clavicle by about ½ in. (1 cm) and can be injured by a penetrating wound above the medial two-thirds of the clavicle. The inferior borders of both lungs are at the following levels: 6th rib in MCL; 8th rib in MAL; 10th rib posteriorly. The pleura follow a similar pattern but the inferior margin is two ribs lower: 8th rib in MCL; 10th rib in MAL;

12th rib posteriorly. A stab wound in the MCL at the level of the 9th rib is likely to puncture the pleura and cause a pneumothorax. However, a deep wound at this point may damage the lung more posteriorly.

11. The pleura.

A. There are three layers of pleura.

B. The whole of the parietal layer of pleura is innervated by the intercostal nerves.

C. The right and left pleural sacs meet in the mid-line at the angle of Louis (T4/T5) and part again inferiorly at the 6th costal cartilage.

D. The costodiaphragmatic recess is an air-filled space.

E. Air in the pleural cavity on one side of the chest is known as a tension pneumothorax.

All false.

There are two layers of pleura: the visceral pleura adjacent to the lung tissue and the parietal pleura adjacent to the diaphragm, pericardium and chest wall. The parietal pleura adjacent to the chest wall is innervated by the intercostal nerves, whereas the parietal pleura adjacent to the diaphragm and pericardium is innervated by the phrenic nerve. Although the pleural sacs meet in the mid-line at the angle of Louis, they diverge at the level of the 4th costal cartilage due to the heart forming the 'cardiac impression' on the left pleural sac. The right pleural sac does, however, continue alone in the mid-line down to the level of the 6th costal cartilage, where it turns laterally to form its inferior margin. The costodiaphragmatic recess is a potential space that allows for expansion of the lung during inspiration. Air in the pleural cavity is known as a pneumothorax. A pneumothorax is referred to as a tension pneumothorax when the causative lesion allows air to enter, but not to escape from, the pleural cavity; this results in displacement of the mediastinum away from the side of the pneumothorax and can be fatal without immediate needle decompression. Needle decompression involves insertion of a hollow cannula into the pleural cavity above the 3rd rib in the 2nd intercostal space in the MCL.

12. The root of the lung.

A. The vagus nerve passes in front.

B. The main bronchi enter at the level of T4.

C. The azygos vein crosses the right hilum.

D. The pulmonary artery (PA) lies below the pulmonary vein (PV).

E. The bronchial arteries run with the bronchial tree.

True:	C E
False:	A B D

The phrenic nerve runs in front of the root of the lung (*Figure 8*). The main bronchi enter at the level of T5 with the PA above and the PV below. The PA carries deoxygenated blood from the right ventricle (RV), and the PVs carry oxygenated blood back

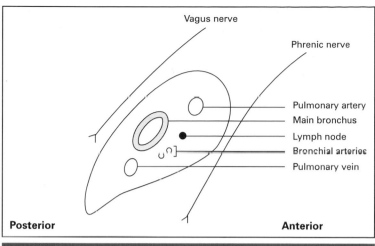

Vagus nerve

Phrenic nerve

Pulmonary artery
Main bronchus
Lymph node
Bronchial arteries
Pulmonary vein

Posterior   **Anterior**

Fig. 8 Cross-section of the lung root, showing the relations of the structures passing through. Note that the phrenic nerve passes in front of the lung root, whereas the vagus nerve passes behind.

to the left atrium (LA). The bronchial arteries run with the bronchial tree and carry oxygenated blood from the descending thoracic aorta to the lung tissue. It is blood from the bronchial arteries which ensures survival of lung tissue when a branch of a PA is occluded by an embolus.

---

13.   The mechanics of breathing.

A.   Contraction of the diaphragm is responsible for the greater part of quiet inspiration.

B.   Expiration is due to contraction of the internal intercostal muscles.

C.   Movement of ribs 2–7 increases the lateral diameter of the chest during inspiration.

D.   Movement of ribs 8–12 increases the antero-posterior diameter of the chest during inspiration.

E.   Transection of the spinal cord at the level of C5 will cause death by respiratory failure.

True:	A
False:	B C D E

Breathing is the term given to movements of the thorax that enable ventilation of the lung tissue. There are two types of breathing: quiet breathing, which occurs at rest; and forced breathing, which occurs during exercise or when there is diseased lung tissue requiring extra ventilation to oxygenate the blood. There are two phases to breathing: inspiration and expiration. During inspiration the thorax expands in three dimensions, i.e., in its vertical, lateral and antero-posterior diameters. This causes the pressure in the pleural cavity to fall to –4 mmHg and therefore air flows into the lungs. During inspiration the thorax expands mainly in its vertical diameter due to contraction and flattening of the hemidiaphragms. This is known as diaphragmatic breathing. Thoracic breathing involves movement of the upper ribs 2–7 in a 'pump-handle' action to increase the antero-posterior diameter of the chest, and the lower ribs 8–12 to move in a 'bucket-handle' manner, thereby increasing the lateral diameter of the chest (see Figure 9). These movements of the ribs are brought about by contraction of the external and internal intercostal muscles.

During quiet breathing, there is a combination of thoracic and diaphragmatic breathing. Thoracic breathing predominates in pregnant women, however, where the bulk of the fetus limits movement of the diaphragm. Conversely, in babies the ribs are mostly horizontal and thoracic breathing is minimal. During forced breathing, accessory muscles of respiration help to expand the thorax. These muscles include the scalene muscles attached to the 1st rib (which is immobile), the pectoral muscles and latissimus dorsi. The pectoral muscles and the latissimus dorsi muscles attach the thoracic cage to the humerus. Thus by fixing the arms (e.g., when athletes bend forward and hold their knees) these muscles help expand the thoracic cage. Elastic recoil of the lungs rather than muscular contractions is responsible for both quiet and forced expiration, although the abdominal muscles may contract in expulsive expiratory efforts such as coughing. Note that transection of the spinal cord at C5 will not necessarily cause death by respiratory failure because, although the intercostal muscles will be paralysed, the phrenic nerve (C3, 4, 5, but mainly C4) will keep the diaphragm alive.

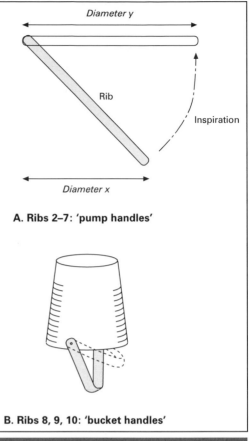

A. Ribs 2–7: 'pump handles'

B. Ribs 8, 9, 10: 'bucket handles'

Fig. 9 Diagram showing how the upper ribs (**A**) and lower ribs (**B**) move to increase the diameter of the thorax (and thereby lower intrathorax pressure).

HEART

14. The embryology of the heart.

A. The coronary arteries are derived from the epicardium.

B. Blood flows through foramen ovale (FO) from right atrium (RA) to LA.

C. There is an interventricular foramen which allows shunting of blood from right to left, thereby bypassing the fetal lungs.

D. The truncus arteriosus is divided into the aorta and pulmonary trunk by a spiral septum.

E. The ductus arteriosus joins the PV to the left ventricle (LV).

True:	A B C D
False:	**E**

The vascular system appears in the middle of the 3rd week of life when the embryo is no longer able to satisfy its nutritional requirements by diffusion alone. Cells with cardiac potential

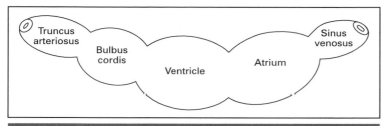

Fig. 10 Representation of the five swellings of the primitive heart tube.

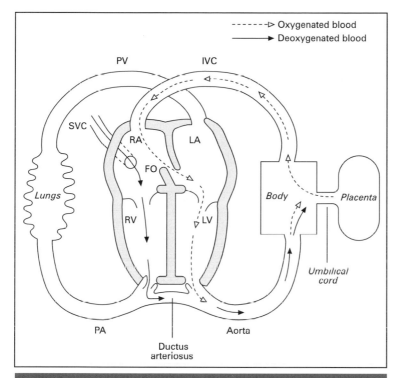

Fig. 11 The fetal circulation. Note that there is little mixing of oxygenated and deoxygenated blood in the right atrium (RA) because blood from the inferior vena cava (IVC) is directed by the IVC valve towards the foramen ovale (FO), and blood from the superior vena cava (SVC) is directed by the SVC valve towards the right ventricle (RV). At birth, the FO and the ductus arteriosus close, redirecting blood towards the lungs. LA = left atrium; LV = left ventricle; PA = pulmonary artery; PV = pulmonary vein.

coalesce into a cardiogenic field and develop into a primitive heart tube. This tube consists of three layers: an outer epicardium; an intervening myocardium; and an inner endocardium. The coronary arteries develop from the epicardium. The heart tube then develops five swellings as shown in *Figure 10*. As the fetus grows, the heart tube folds and twists around upon itself. Septa form across the primitive ventricle and atrium leaving foramina for the right-to-left shunting of blood to bypass the as yet non-functional lung. The FO lies between the atria, and the interventricular foramen between the ventricles. The interventricular foramen eventually disappears and the ductus arteriosus acts as a lung-bypass shunt between the pulmonary trunk and the aorta. The ductus arteriosus closes at birth when the new-born baby takes its first breath; it persists as the ligamentum arteriosum. A simplified diagram of the fetal circulation is shown in *Figure 11*.

15. The pericardium and borders of the heart.

A. The heart is enclosed in three layers of pericardium.

B. The right heart border is formed entirely from RA.

C. The apex is the most inferior and most lateral part of the heart.

D.   The surface markings of the heart valves are important for auscultation of the heart sounds.

E.   The fibrous skeleton of the heart consists of four rings to which the musculature of the chambers is attached.

True:	A B
False:	C D E

There are three layers of pericardium, a fibrous layer and two serous layers. The fibrous layer is conical and surrounds the heart and the roots of the great vessels. Inside the fibrous layer, is the serous pericardium, which has a parietal and visceral layer. The parietal layer is in contact with the fibrous pericardium, and it becomes the visceral layer as it twists round the roots of the great vessels to lie against the heart surface. This creates two pericardial grooves: the oblique sinus between the IVC and the four PVs; and the transverse sinus, which separates the SVC and LA from the pulmonary trunk and aorta.

The right heart border is entirely RA, the left border mainly LV with a small contribution from the LA, and the inferior border chiefly RV with some RA and some LV. The front of the heart is mainly RV, the back of the heart is mainly LA, and the inferior surface of the heart is made up of RV and LV.

The heart can loosely be represented as a fist held in front of the sternum. The right heart border runs from the lower edge of the third costal cartilage to the lower border of the 6th costal cartilage just to the right of the sternum. The left heart border runs from the lower border of the second costal cartilage, about ¾ in. (2 cm) to the left of the sternum, down to the apex in the 5th intercostal space, about 3½ in. (9 cm) from the mid-line. The heart valves lie in a near vertical line behind the sternum in the order: pulmonary valve (highest), aortic, mitral and tricuspid (lowest). The heart sounds are best heard where the valve's respective chamber lies closest to the chest wall. For the mitral valve, this is over the apex beat. The tricuspid is best heard just to the right of the lower sternum, the pulmonary in the left third intercostal space, and the aortic in the right second intercostal space.

The skeleton of the heart consists of a pair of fibrous rings joined to form a figure-8 at the atrioventricular orifices.

16.   The right atrium.

A.   The coronary sinus opens between the IVC and the tricuspid valve (TV).

B.   The sinoatrial node (SAN) lies in the auricle.

C.   The RA receives the anterior cardiac veins.

D.   The entire inner surface of the RA is roughened by musculae pectinatae.

E.   The fossa ovalis may be patent in the normal subject.

True:	A C E
False:	B D

The RA is shown in *Figure 12*. A good *aide-memoire* is to remember that there are six 'openings' in the RA: the SVC and IVC; the TV; the coronary sinus; the fossa ovalis; and the anterior cardiac veins (up to four of them). The fossa ovalis, a remnant of the FO, is not always a true opening but it is probe-patent in 10% of normal subjects, i.e., it is possible to pass an instrument, such as dissecting forceps, through to the LA. The auricle of the RA is a remnant of the primitive atrium and has a roughened surface due to muscular folds known as the musculae pectinatae. The crista terminalis forms the boundary between the auricle and the smooth wall of the rest of the RA. The crista terminalis can be identified on the external surface of the heart by a groove known as the sulcus terminalis. The SAN lies in the upper end of the crista terminalis, while the

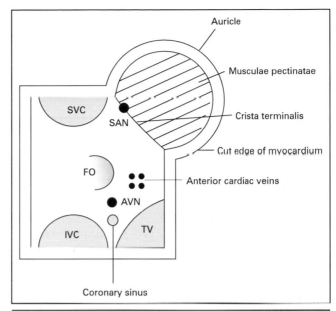

Fig. 12 Diagrammatic representation of the right atrium, showing the atrium cut open anteriorly, with the auricle folded out to show its inner surface. The six 'openings' in the atrium are shown: superior vena cava (SVC); inferior vena cava (IVC); foramen ovale (FO); tricuspid valve (TV); coronary sinus; and anterior cardiac veins. Note the location of the sinoatrial node (SAN) in the crista terminalis, and of the atrioventricular node (AVN) just anterior to the coronary sinus.

atrioventricular node (AVN) is found lower down in the chamber, near the opening of the IVC. The smooth-walled part of the RA is derived from the primitive sinus venosus.

It is useful to remember the following adult derivatives of the primitive heart tube swellings:

Truncus arteriosus

- Aorta and pulmonary trunk: formed as the truncus is divided by a spiral septum (hence the spiral relation of these two vessels).

- Infundibulum of the ventricles: the smooth-walled part of the adult ventricles.

Sinus venosus

- The smooth-walled part of the main chambers of the atria.

Primitive atrium

- The rough-surfaced auricles of the adult atria.

Primitive ventricle

- The rough-walled contractile part of the adult ventricles.

Note: The LA shows the same internal structure as the RA and also has six 'openings': the mitral valve; the four PVs (two left and two right); and the fossa ovalis. However, there is no SAN or AVN in the LA.

17. The right ventricle.

A. The papillary muscle contracts to open the TV.

B. The infundibulum is a remnant of the truncus arteriosus of the primitive heart tube.

C. Each cusp of the TV is attached to a single papillary muscle *via* chordae tendinae.

D. The trabeculae carneae cover the entire inner surface.

E. The moderator band carries conducting tissue.

True:	B E
False:	A C D

The RV is shown diagrammatically in *Figure 13*. The chamber is divided into an upper non-contractile smooth part, known as the infundibulum (derived from the truncus arteriosus), and a lower contractile zone. The contractile part is covered by muscular folds known as trabeculae carneae. Three of these

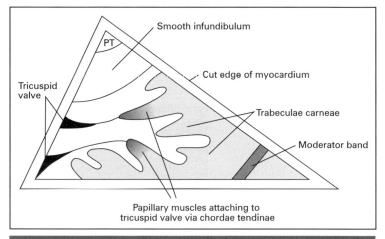

Fig. 13 Diagrammatic representation of the right ventricle. The anterior wall has been cut away to reveal a triangular chamber with a smooth upper part (infundibulum).

trabeculae carneae are specialised papillary muscles which connect *via* chordae tendinae to the cusps of the TV (each cusp is connected to two papillary muscles). The papillary muscles prevent the cusps from folding back into the RA during contraction of the ventricles but have no role in opening of the TV. The moderator band runs perpendicular to the trabeculae carneae and carries the right branch of the atrioventricular bundle of conducting tissue.

18. The chambers of the heart.

A. The RA contains the SAN.

B. The papillary muscles of the RV give off chordae tendinae to the tricuspid and pulmonary valves.

C. The LA is muscular walled, apart from a smooth area known as the fossa ovalis.

D. The mitral valve has two equal-sized cusps.

E. The muscle walls of the LV are five times as thick as those of the RV.

True:	A
False:	B C D E

The RA receives deoxygenated blood from the rest of the body. Its inferior surface is almost entirely the opening of the IVC. The SVC empties into the superior part, but here, to the left, lies the muscular right atrial appendage. At the angle between the two lies the start of a groove called the sulcus terminalis. At the top of this can be found the pacemaker of the heart, a knot of tissue known as the SAN. The AVN lies lower down in the interatrial septum, near where the coronary sinus drains.

The RV has muscular walls known as trabeculae carneae, with strips of muscle known as the papillary muscle. These papillary muscles attach to the cusps of the TV *via* chordae tendinae to keep the valve closed during ventricular systole when the pulmonary valve is open.

The LA, like the RA, has a muscular appendage as well as its smooth-walled part formed from the four PVs. As in the RA, a small hollow area can be seen at dissection. This is the fossa ovalis and is the remnant of the primary septum closing off the foramen ovale. The mitral valve lies between the LA and ventricle. It has two cusps, the anterior being larger and thicker than the posterior. Like the tricuspid, it is held shut during ventricular systole by chordae tendinae. The LV has a muscle wall which is three times as thick as the RV wall, enabling it to generate more than five times the pressure.

19. The coronary arteries.

A. Both the right and left coronary arteries travel in the atrioventricular grooves.

B. Both right and left coronary arteries give off interventricular branches.

C. Only the right coronary artery (RCA) gives off a marginal branch.

D. The left coronary artery (LCA) passes behind the pulmonary trunk.

E. There is significant anastomosis between the right and left coronary arteries.

True:	A B D
False:	C E

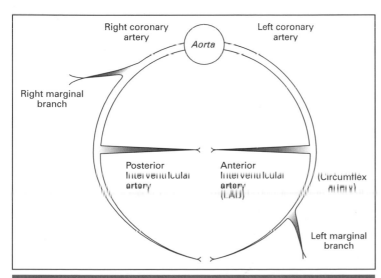

Fig. 14 Diagram summarising the branches of the coronary arteries and how they anastomose. Shaded areas show branches of the main arteries; the unshaded areas are the arteries proper. LAD = left anterior descending artery.

In simple terms, RCA and LCA run in opposite directions from the aorta, around the atrioventricular groove of the heart, to meet each other at the back where they form a very weak anastomosis. Both give off two corresponding branches: interventricular branches and marginal branches. The anterior interventricular artery (AIVA) comes from the LCA and is the largest branch of the coronary arteries; it runs in the anterior interventricular groove to make a weak anastomosis at the apex of the heart with the posterior interventricular artery (PIVA), a branch of the RCA. Prior to giving off the PIVA, the RCA gives off a marginal branch, the right marginal artery (RMA), which runs across the RV. In contrast, the LCA gives off the left marginal artery (LMA), which runs over the LV, after it has given rise to the AIVA. This simple system of nomenclature is confused by the clinician's use of the terms left anterior descending artery (LAD) and circumflex artery. The LAD refers to the AIVA and the circumflex artery refers to the continuation of the LCA after the LAD (circumflex refers to the bend in the course of the LCA after it emerges from behind the pulmonary trunk and passes behind the heart). A diagrammatic representation of the coronary arteries is shown in *Figure 14*.

20. The venous drainage of the heart.

A. The coronary sinus opens into the RA near the SVC.

B. The great cardiac vein runs with the left anterior descending branch of the LCA.

C. The anterior cardiac veins drain into the RV.

D. The small cardiac vein drains into the coronary sinus.

E. There are no veins entering the LV.

True:	B D
False:	A C E

The heart has a dual venous drainage: two-thirds drain *via* the coronary sinus and anterior cardiac veins into the RA; and one-third drains directly into all the chambers of the heart *via* the small venae cordis minimae. The coronary sinus opens in the inferior part of the RA between the opening of the IVC and the TV. The coronary sinus receives the following branches.

• Great cardiac vein: runs in the anterior atrioventricular groove with LAD.

• Middle cardiac vein: runs in the inferior atrioventricular groove.

• Small cardiac vein: runs with the RMA.

• Oblique vein: descends obliquely across the posterior aspect of the LA.

There are approximately 3–4 anterior cardiac veins, and they all cross the anterior interventricular groove and open into the RA.

21. The vessels of the heart.

A. The RCA arises from the right posterior aortic sinus.

B. The LCA arises from the left posterior coronary sinus.

C. The circumflex branch of the LCA supplies the SAN in 40% of hearts.

D. The LAD supplies the anterior walls of both ventricles.

E. The great cardiac vein runs with the LAD before it empties into the RA.

True:	B C D
False:	A E

The blood supply to the heart is provided by the right and left coronary arteries, which are branches off the ascending aorta. The RCA comes off the anterior aortic sinus and emerges from behind the right atrial appendage to run down in the atrioventricular groove. It reaches the back of the heart in the posterior interventricular groove. The right coronary supplies the SAN in 60% of all hearts. The main branch off the right coronary is called the marginal artery; it runs across the inferior border of the heart to supply the RV.

The LCA arises from the left posterior aortic sinus. It emerges from behind the left atrial appendage and gives off a large branch, which runs down the anterior interventricular groove to supply both ventricles. This is the LAD and is often affected by disease. The continuation of the LCA is actually narrower than this branch. It is called the circumflex artery and runs around to reach the back of the heart, supplying the SAN in about 40% of cases. It should be appreciated that, although the above description is the most common arrangement, there is anatomical variation.

The coronary sinus is the main venous drainage of the heart and receives blood from the great, middle and small cardiac veins, the oblique vein and the posterior vein of the LV. The great cardiac vein runs with the LAD, the middle cardiac vein with the PIVA, and the small cardiac vein with the marginal artery. The anterior cardiac veins run across the RV and drain directly into the RA. There are also venae cordis minimae, tiny veins in all four chambers that open directly into their respective chambers.

22. The heart valves.

A. Closure of the mitral and tricuspid valves is responsible for the 2nd heart sound.

B. The semilunar valves are bicuspid.

C. The aortic valve has a single posterior cusp.

D. The pulmonary valve has a single anterior cusp.

E. The mitral valve has three cusps.

All false.

The mitral valve has two cusps (bicuspid), and lies between the LA and LV; and the TV (three cusps) lies between the RA and RV. Their closure forms the 1st heart sound while the 2nd heart sound is due to closure of the aortic and pulmonary valves. The aortic and pulmonary valves both have three semilunar-shaped (half-moon-shaped) cusps. The aortic valve has a single anterior cusp and two posterior cusps, whereas the pulmonary valve has a single posterior cusp and two anterior cusps. This can easily be remembered as follows: aorta begins with a single letter A and has one anterior cusp and pulmonary begins with a single P and has one posterior cusp. *Figure 15*

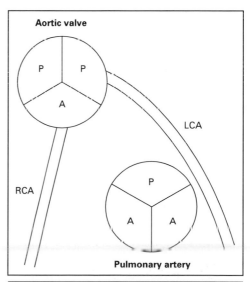

Fig. 15 Diagrammatic representation of the aorta and pulmonary trunk, as seen from above, to show the arrangement of the valves. Note that the aortic valve has a single anterior cusp (A) and the pulmonary valve a single posterior cusp (P). The left coronary artery (LCA) passes posterior to the pulmonary trunk. RCA = right coronary artery.

shows the aortic and pulmonary valves as seen from above (i.e., with the aorta and pulmonary trunk cut through). Note how the LCA passes behind the pulmonary trunk.

23. The conducting system of the heart.

A. The SAN is situated in the crista terminalis of the RA.

B. The AVN is situated in the RA, posterior to the opening of the coronary sinus.

C. The atrioventricular bundle of His is the only muscular connection between the atria and the ventricles.

D. The septomarginal trabecula (moderate band) is found in the LV.

E. The SAN receives its blood supply from the LCA.

True:	A C
False:	B D E

The SAN is the pacemaker of the heart and it receives its blood supply from the RCA. Myocardial action potentials are sent from the SAN through the atria to the AVN. From the AVN, the bundle of His transmits electrical signals to the interventricular septum and through the right and left crus to the respective ventricles. The bundle of His is a group of modified myocardial fibres and provides the only muscular connection between the atria and the ventricles, which are otherwise separated by the fibrous skeleton of the heart. The right crus is visible in the RV as the septomarginal trabecula (moderate band) which connects to the anterior papillary muscles. The function of the conducting system of the heart is to ensure the coordinated contraction of the chambers. Subendocardial Purkinje fibres ensure that the ventricles start to contract at their apices.

NERVES OF THE THORAX

24. The vagus nerves.

A. The right vagus nerve pierces the diaphragm in front of the oesophagus.

B. The vagus nerves run in front of the root of the lung.

C. The right recurrent laryngeal nerve is a thoracic branch of the right vagus nerve.

D. The only function of the vagus nerves in the thorax is to carry parasympathetic innervation to the heart.

E. The recurrent laryngeal nerves supply all the intrinsic muscles of the larynx.

All false.

The vagus nerves (cranial nerves X) arise in the medulla and exit the skull through the jugular foramina. They pass down through the neck in the carotid sheath into the thorax in front of the great arteries. Both vagi pass behind the root of the lung and onto the oesophagus where they form the oesophageal plexus. The right vagus passes posteriorly, and the left vagus anteriorly, to the oesophagus; in this position they pass through the diaphragm to supply the stomach. The vagi contribute to the pulmonary and cardiac plexus in the thorax. The latter is found in front of the bifurcation of the trachea and receives sympathetic fibres from T1–T4 as well as the parasympathetic fibres from the vagi. The left recurrent laryngeal nerve branches from the left vagus as it passes over the arch of the aorta and then hooks back up under the ligamentum arteriosum (remnant of the ductus arteriosus). The right recurrent laryngeal nerve, however, is not a thoracic structure, as it hooks around the right subclavian artery in the neck. The recurrent laryngeal nerves supply all the intrinsic muscles of the larynx except cricothyroid, which is supplied by the external laryngeal branch of the vagus nerve.

25.   The phrenic nerves.

A.   Arise from the posterior rami of C3, 4, 5.

B.   Run in front of the root of the lung.

C.   Are mixed motor and sensory nerves.

D.   Do not provide any innervation to abdominal structures.

E.   The right phrenic nerve leaves the thorax with the IVC.

True:	B C E
False:	A D

The phrenic nerves arise from the anterior rami of C3, 4, 5 and provide motor innervation to the diaphragm (mnemonic: 3, 4, 5 keeps the diaphragm alive) and carry sensory output from the diaphragmatic and mediastinal pleura, the pericardium and the diaphragmatic peritoneum. The roots of C3, 4, 5 also supply the skin over the shoulder, and pain from the phrenic nerve may be felt as referred shoulder pain. The right phrenic nerve descends through the thorax on the 'venous' border of the heart and vessels, running, respectively, to the right of the right brachiocephalic vein, the SVC, the RA, and the IVC with which it passes through the diaphragm. The left phrenic nerve, on the other hand, passes on the 'arterial' border of the heart and vessels, running respectively to the left of the left subclavian artery, the aortic arch, and the LV, before piercing the diaphragm alone. Both phrenic nerves pass in front of the lung roots.

26.   The thoracic sympathetic trunk.

A.   The thoracic sympathetic trunk runs down anterior to the heads of all the 12 ribs.

B.   The first thoracic sympathetic ganglion joins the inferior cervical ganglion to form the stellate ganglion.

C.   The thoracic sympathetic trunk lies anterior to the thoracic duct.

D.   Sympathetic fibres supply the heart, great vessels, lungs, pleura, oesophagus and skin.

E.   The splanchnic nerves lie lateral to the sympathetic trunk.

True:	B
False:	A C D E

The sympathetic chain in the thorax descends from the cervical chain along the neck of the 1st rib, along the heads of the 2nd–10th ribs, and over the bodies of the 11th and 12th thoracic vertebrae. The sympathetic ganglion at T1 usually joins the inferior cervical

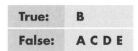

ganglion to form the stellate ganglion. The thoracic duct lies anterior to the trunk and has only the vertebrae behind as a posterior relation. Sympathetic fibres, with the thoracic spinal nerves, are distributed to the skin of the thoracic wall, and post-ganglionic fibres (T1–T5) are distributed to the heart, great vessels, lungs and oesophagus. The pleura have no autonomic innervation. The intercostal nerves segmentally innervate the parietal pleura. The splanchnic nerves, greater (T5–T10), lesser (T10–T11) and least (T12), are preganglionic sympathetic fibres which lie medial to the sympathetic trunk on the bodies of the thoracic vertebrae, and traverse the diaphragm to enter the abdomen where they synapse and are distributed to the abdominal viscera.

SUPERIOR AND POSTERIOR MEDIASTINUM

27.   The contents of the superior mediastinum.

A.   The thymus is the most anterior.

B.   The trachea lies anterior to the oesophagus.

C.   The right recurrent laryngeal nerve lies anterior to the oesophagus.

D.   The great veins lie behind the branches of the aortic arch.

E.   The thoracic duct lies posterior to the oesophagus.

True:	A B C
False:	D E

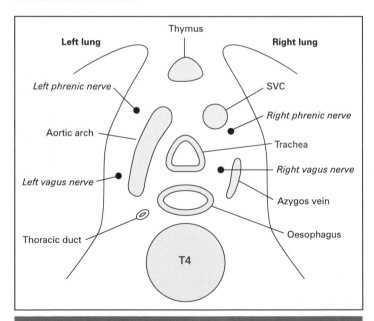

Fig. 16 Transverse section of the superior mediastinum at T4, showing relations of the enclosed structures. SVC = superior vena cava.

Figure 16 shows the relations of structures in the superior mediastinum (see also Figure 1). Note that the right recurrent laryngeal nerve is not shown, because it is not a thoracic structure.

28. The great vessels.

A. The jugular veins drain directly into the SVC.

B. The left subclavian vein (LSCV) and the internal jugular vein (IJV) join to form the left brachiocephalic vein behind the sternoclavicular joint.

C. The left brachiocephalic vein crosses all the branches of the aortic arch.

D. The left common carotid artery (LCCA) and the left subclavian artery arise from the left brachiocephalic trunk (LBCT).

True:	B C
False:	A D

The great vessels (*Figure 17*) of the superior mediastinum all carry blood to and from the arms and the head. There is, therefore, one great artery and one great vein for each arm, and one of each for both sides of the head. The subclavian veins and the IJV drain to the SVC through their confluence into the right and left brachiocephalic (innominate) veins. However, there is only a single brachiocephalic arterial trunk on the right, giving rise to the right common carotid artery (RCCA) and the left subclavian artery. The LCCA and subclavian arteries arise directly from the aortic arch.

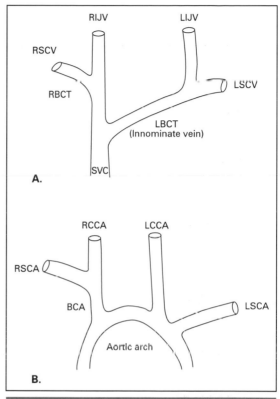

Fig. 17 A. The great veins: superior vena cava (SVC); right internal jugular vein (RIJV); left internal jugular vein (LIJV); right subclavian vein (RSCV); and left subclavian vein (LSCV). LBCT = left brachiocephalic trunk; RBCT = right brachiocephalic trunk. **B.** The great arteries: brachiocephalic artery (BCA); right common carotid artery (RCCA); left common carotid artery (LCCA); right subclavian artery (RSCA); and left subclavian artery (LSCA).

29. The descending thoracic aorta.

A Begins to the right of the vertebral column.

B Is a mid-line structure at the level of T8.

C. Is crossed by the oesophagus inferiorly.

D. Gives rise to 11 posterior intercostal arteries and the subcostal artery.

E. Passes through the diaphragm at T10.

True:	B C
False:	A D E

The descending thoracic aorta starts to the left of the body of T5 as a continuation of the aortic arch. It has become a mid-line structure by the time it reaches T8 and is crossed inferiorly by the oesophagus before it passes behind the crura of the diaphragm at T12. It gives rise to nine pairs of posterior intercostal arteries (3rd–11th intercostal spaces) and the subcostal artery (the 1st and 2nd intercostal arteries are branches of the costocervical trunk from the subclavian artery). The right posterior intercostal arteries from T3 to T8 cross the mid-line as they arise from the left sided descending aorta. The thoracic aorta also gives rise to the bronchial arteries and branches to the oesophagus.

30. The azygos and hemiazygos veins.

A. The azygos system drains all the intercostal spaces *via* the posterior intercostal veins.

B. The hemiazygos system drains into the azygos vein.

C. The azygos vein drains into the SVC.

D. The hemiazygos vein drains into the IVC.

E. The azygos vein may pass through the diaphragm with the aorta.

True:	B C E
False:	A D

On the right side of the thorax, the azygos vein drains blood from the 5th to 11th posterior intercostal veins directly, and from the 2nd to 4th posterior intercostal veins indirectly, *via* the right superior intercostal vein. On the left, the hemiazygos vein drains the thoracic wall in a similar fashion, except that the left superior intercostal vein drains into the left brachiocephalic vein. Blood from the 1st intercostal space drains into the brachiocephalic veins *via* the highest posterior intercostal veins.

31. The thoracic oesophagus.

A. The LA is an anterior relation.

B. The thoracic oesophagus pierces the diaphragm at T8.

C. The right bronchus constricts the thoracic oesophagus.

D. Branches of the internal thoracic artery supply the thoracic oesophagus.

E. The thoracic oesophagus is part innervated by the phrenic nerves.

True:	A
False:	B C D E

The thoracic oesophagus has the trachea, left bronchus and LA as anterior relations in the inferior mediastinum. Subsequently, it is possible for a dilated LA (commonly associated with valvular heart disease) to displace the oesophagus posteriorly and, if severe, to constrict it. Blood supply in the thoracic region is derived from the thoracic aorta and the veins drain into the azygos system. Both vagi form a plexus of parasympathetic innervation, encompassing the oesophagus. The IVC and right phrenic nerve pierce the diaphragm at T8; the vagi, left gastric vessels and oesophagus at T10; and the descending aorta, azygos vein and thoracic duct at T12. The phrenic nerve (remember, C3, 4, 5 keeps the diaphragm alive!) principally arises from C4. It is both motor to and sensory from the diaphragm, and sensory from the pleura and fibrous pericardium.

32. The thoracic duct.

A. Drains lymph from the right side of the head.

B. Lies posterior to the oesophagus at T4.

C. Traverses the diaphragm at T10.

D. Usually drains into the left internal jugular vein (LIJV).

E. Is a continuation of the cisterna chyli.

True:	E
False:	A B C D

The thoracic duct is a continuation of the cisterna chyli in the abdomen as it traverses the diaphragm at T12 along with the aorta and azygos vein. It drains the abdomen, and lower limbs, and is joined by lymphatics draining the left side of the head and neck before it drains into the left brachiocephalic vein. On the right side of the head and neck, lymph drains into the right lymphatic duct *via* subclavian and jugular trunks before joining the mediastinal trunk which then drains into the right brachiocephalic vein. The thoracic duct lies as a posterior relation to the oesophagus for most of its journey in the thorax, until it crosses to the left of it at the level of T5. The angle of Louis (T4/T5) is an extremely important landmark, with many important points of anatomy occurring at this point.

- Arch of the aorta: commences, and the descending aorta begins.

- Thoracic duct: goes from posterior to the left of the oesophagus.

- Azygos vein: joins the SVC at T4.

- Level of the 2nd costal cartilage, angle of Louis, sternal angle: important for accurate location of rib numbers and intercostal spaces.

- Brachiocephalic veins: join to form the SVC.

- Trachea: bifurcates into L and R main bronchi.

2. Abdomen

TOPIC CHECK LIST

ABDOMINAL WALLS AND PERITONEUM

1. The abdominal regions.

A. The subcostal plane is at the level L3 (10th rib).

B. The lateral planes are not the same as the MCL.

C. The lateral planes pass through the inguinal ligament.

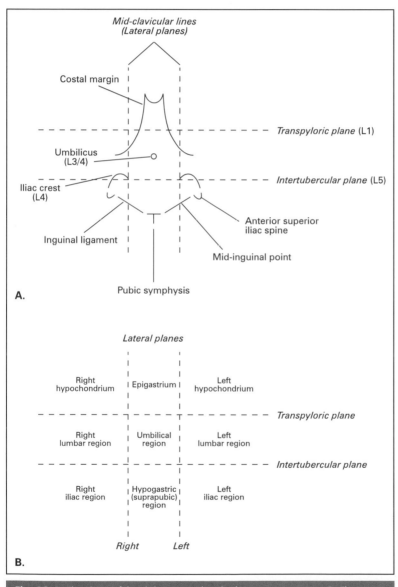

Fig. 18 A. The planes of the abdomen, used to divide it into nine regions. **B.** The names of the nine abdominal regions.

D.   The umbilical region is defined above by the subcostal plane and below by the supracrestal plane.

E.   The hypochondrium lies just above the pubic symphysis.

True:	C
False:	**A B D E**

The abdomen can be divided into nine regions by the following planes: lateral planes; transpyloric plane (L1); intertubercular plane (L5, level of iliac tubercles). The lateral planes are the same as the MCL and pass through the mid-inguinal point (half-way between the anterior superior iliac spine (ASIS) of the iliac crest and the pubic symphysis). The regions and their names are shown in *Figure 18* projected onto an outline of the bony boundaries of the abdomen presented at the bottom of the figure.

2.   The surface anatomy of the abdomen.

A.   The transpyloric plane of Addison lies at the level of the xiphoid.

B.   The tip of the gallbladder lies at the level of the 9th costal cartilage.

C.   The highest point of the liver lies at the level of the nipples.

D.   The neck of the pancreas is palpable at the level of L1 in the mid-line.

E.   The right kidney is lower than the left kidney.

True:	B C E
False:	**A D**

The transpyloric plane of Addison lies half-way between the suprasternal notch and the pubis at the level of L1, i.e., approximately a hand's breadth below the xiphoid. The only palpable organs in the normal abdomen are the aorta and the lower pole of the right kidney. Important surface markings of the abdominal viscera are as follows:

* Liver: nipple line superiorly, 10th rib inferiorly.
* Gallbladder: tip lies at 9th costal cartilage in the MCL.
* Kidney: superior pole at 12th rib posteriorly (right slightly lower than left).
* Spleen: 9th, 10th and 11th ribs posteriorly.
* Pancreas: neck at L1.

3.   The transpyloric plane of Addison.

The following structures lie in the transpyloric plane of Addison:

A.   The fundus of the stomach.

B.   The coeliac trunk.

C.   Renal pelvis.

D.   Termination of the spinal cord.

E.   9th rib.

True:	C D E
False:	**A B**

The following structures lie in the transpyloric plane of Addison (L1):

- Pylorus of the stomach
- Fundus of the gallbladder
- 9th rib
- Superior mesenteric artery (SMA)
- Neck of the pancreas
- Renal pelvis
- Termination of the spinal cord

4. The fascia of the anterior abdominal wall.

A. The deep fascia of the abdominal wall is continuous with that of the trunk.

B. Camper's fascia is continuous with the rest of the body.

C. Scarpa's fascia is thickest above the umbilicus.

D. Scarpa's fascia joins the fascia lata of the lower limb.

E. Colle's fascia is deep to the fascia transversalis.

True:	B D
False:	A C E

There is no deep fascia on the trunk. Camper's fascia is the outer fatty layer of superficial fascia, and is continuous with the superficial fascia of the rest of the body. Scarpa's fascia is the deeper fibrous layer of superficial fascia; it is thickest below the umbilicus and joins with the fascia lata in the thigh, forming the 'swimming trunk' pattern shown in *Figure 19*. Colle's fascia is the perineal extension of Scarpa's fascia. The fascia transversalis lies intra-abdominally outwith the peritoneum, next to the transversus abdominis muscle (TAM).

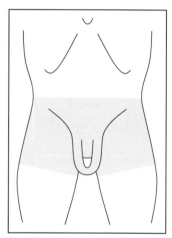

Fig. 19 Scarpa's fascia. Note the 'swimming trunk' distribution.

5. The anterior abdominal wall muscles.

A. External oblique interdigitates with serratus anterior.

B. TAM has an origin from the inferior aspect of the costal margin.

C. NV structures run between external oblique and internal oblique muscles.

D. RAM has three transverse tendinous intersections which lie above the level of the umbilicus.

E. The rectus sheath is deficient posteriorly only below the umbilicus.

True:	A D
False:	B C E

The finger-like fibres of serratus anterior attach to the upper eight ribs (ribs 1–8). The lower fibres of serratus anterior interdigitate with the costal origin of EOM which attaches to the

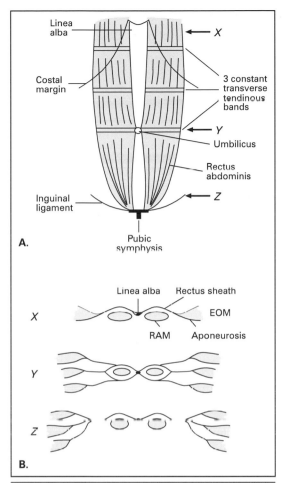

Fig. 20 A. Rectus abdominis muscle (RAM) seen from the front. **B.** Cross-section of RAM at points *X*, *Y* and *Z*, as indicated in **A**, showing how the rectus sheath is formed by aponeuroses of the external oblique muscle (EOM), the internal oblique muscle (IOM) and the transversus abdominis muscle (TAM). Note how the rectus sheath is incomplete superiorly (*X*) and inferiorly (*Z*).

lower eight ribs (ribs 5–12). Both the internal oblique muscle (IOM) and TAM have origins from the iliac crest, thoracolumbar fascia and ribs. Nerves, arteries and veins run between IOM and TAM: this is analogous to the thoracic NV plane, where the NV bundles run between the second and third intercostal muscle layers. RAM has three constant transverse tendinous intersections above the umbilicus, and occasionally a fourth below. The rectus sheath, formed by the aponeuroses of EOM, IOM and TAM, is free posteriorly below the umbilicus, but also superiorly at the level of the xiphoid process (*Figure 20*).

6.	**The blood supply of the anterior abdominal wall.**

A.   The normal direction of arterial blood flow is away from the umbilicus.

B.   The inferior epigastric artery lies superficial to the inguinal ligament.

C. The superficial epigastric artery is a branch of the external iliac artery.

D. The axillary vein receives venous blood from the anterior abdominal wall.

E. The hemiazygos system is not involved in its venous drainage.

True:	D
False:	A B C E

The direction of arterial blood flow is towards, and the direction of venous flow away from, the umbilicus. The blood supply of the anterior abdominal wall can be divided into superficial and deep components: these are shown diagrammatically in *Figure 21*. Notice that in both divisions there is a vertical and horizontal component. The horizontal superficial vessels are, in fact, superficial branches of the deep horizontal vessels given off in the MAL. The superficial vessels, including the vertically placed lateral thoracic vessels (from the axillary vessels) and superficial epigastric vessels (from the femoral vessels), run in the superficial fascia. The lumbar veins drain posteriorly into the IVC. There is, however, a connection with the ascending lumbar veins through which blood may bypass to the azygos and hemiazygos systems.

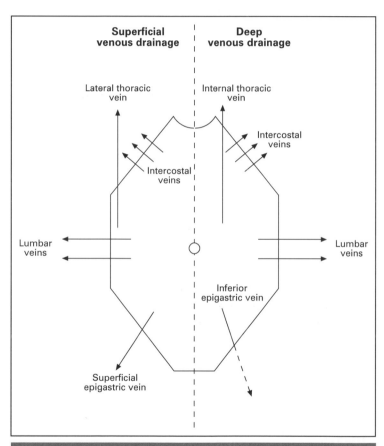

Fig. 21 Venous drainage of the anterior abdominal wall. Superficial drainage is shown on the left side of the diagram, and deep drainage on the right.

7. The innervation of the anterior abdominal wall.

A. The 10th intercostal nerve supplies the skin over the umbilicus.

B. The lower seven intercostal nerves and the subcostal nerve (T5–T12) supply the muscles of the anterior abdominal wall.

C. Rectus femoris receives innervation from L1.

D. The nerves supplying the anterior abdominal wall run between IOM and TAM.

E. The ilioinguinal nerve supplies the cremaster muscle.

True:	A D
False:	B C E

The anterior abdominal wall muscles are supplied by the lower six intercostal nerves (T6–T11) and the subcostal nerve (T12). In addition, all the muscles attached to the iliac crest receive innervation from L1 through the iliohypogastric and ilioinguinal nerves. The cremaster muscle, an extension of the IOM to the scrotum, is innervated by L1 through the genito-femoral nerve. The nerves run between the inner two layers of muscle in the same way as in the intercostal nerves in the thorax. Important skin dermatomes to remember are:

- Xiphoid T6

- Umbilicus T10

- Suprapubic L1

8. Lymphatic drainage of the anterior abdominal wall.

A. Lymph drains in an almost quadrantic manner, i.e., the four quadrants around the umbilicus drain to different lymph nodes.

B. There are no nodes in the anterior abdominal wall.

C. Above the umbilicus, lymph drains to the deep axillary nodes.

D. Below the umbilicus, lymph drains to the superficial inguinal nodes.

E. An inflammatory lesion to the right of the mid-line below the umbilicus may cause left superficial inguinal lymphadenopathy.

All true.

Lymphatic drainage of the anterior abdominal wall occurs in a quadrantic manner (shown in *Figure 22*). The only exception to this is that, while above the umbilicus lymph does not cross the mid-line, below the umbilicus lymph near the mid-line may drain to both sides.

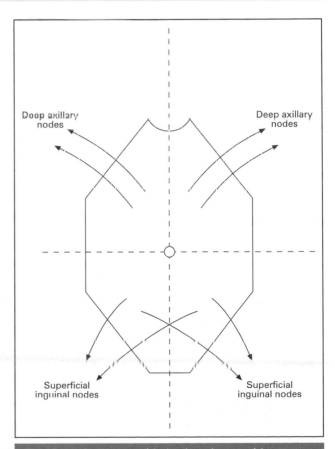

Fig. 22 Quadrantic nature of the lymphatic drainage of the anterior abdominal wall. Note how the drainage crosses the mid-line, below the umbilicus.

9.   The inguinal canal.

A.   The internal ring lies at the mid-point of the inguinal ligament.

B.   A direct inguinal hernia comes through the internal ring.

C.   The anterior boundary of the canal is formed by the inguinal ligament.

D.   The lateral part of the posterior boundary of the canal is formed by the conjoint tendon.

E.   The external ring lies above, and medial to, the pubic tubercle.

True:	A E
False:	B C D

The mid-inguinal point and the mid-point of the inguinal ligament are different. The mid-point of the inguinal ligament lies half-way between the ASIS and the pubic tubercle. The internal (deep) ring lies just above this point. The mid-inguinal point is ¾ in. (1.5 cm) higher, half-way between the ASIS and the pubic symphysis; this is the position of the femoral artery. The inferior epigastric artery marks the medial border of the internal ring. Direct inguinal hernias push through the posterior border of the inguinal canal medial to the artery. Indirect inguinal hernias pass through the internal ring lateral to the artery. A frequently asked question concerns the boundaries of the inguinal canal. The anterior wall is the aponeurosis of the external oblique, reinforced laterally by the IOM. The posterior wall is formed by the conjoint tendon medially, while laterally it is only transversalis fascia. Inferiorly lies the inguinal ligament (remember the rotated position of the pelvis). Above, fibres of IOM and TAM arch over. The external ring lies medial to the pubic tubercle; hernias below and lateral to the pubic tubercle are, by definition, femoral.

10.   The spermatic cord.

A.   Contains three layers of fascia.

B.   Carries lymphatics which drain the testis into inguinal lymph nodes.

C.   Contains the processus vaginalis.

D.   Carries the cremasteric artery.

E.   Has the iliohypogastric nerve lying on it.

True:	A C D
False:	B E

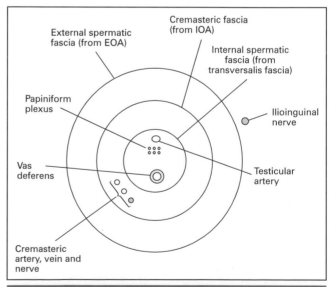

Fig. 23 Cross-section of the spermatic cord. EOA = external oblique aponeurosis; IOA = internal oblique aponeurosis.

The structure of the spermatic cord, a cross-section of which is presented in *Figure 23*, can be understood by following the descent of the testis from the abdomen, where it is formed in fetal life, down to its final destination in the scrotum. It drags with it three layers of fascia from the muscle layers through which it pushes. The internal spermatic fascia is acquired as the testis pushes through the fascia transversalis at the internal ring; the cremasteric fascia, including the cremasteric muscle fibres, is acquired from the IOM layer; and the external spermatic fascia is formed as the testis passes through the external ring. These three layers continue to be represented in the three coverings of the testis. The processus vaginalis is a remnant of the embryological descent; when patent, it can form the sac of an indirect hernia. The blood supply to the testis is the testicular artery. This comes off the aorta at the level of the original position of the testis, at around L1. The lymph drainage of the testis follows the blood supply and so drains into para-aortic nodes. Two other arteries are found in the spermatic cord: the cremasteric artery, which is a branch of the inferior epigastric artery; and the artery to the vas, which is a branch of the inferior vesical artery. Other contents of the spermatic cord are the pampiniform venous plexus, sympathetics, the vas deferens itself, and the genital branch of the genito-femoral nerve. The ilio-inguinal nerve lies on top of the cord, where it can be anaesthetised prior to hernia surgery, hence anaesthetising the skin of the overlying groin.

11. The posterior abdominal wall.

A. Psoas major attaches to the vertebral bodies of the lumbar vertebrae.

B. Quadratus lumborum attaches to the 12th rib above, the iliac crest below, and the transverse processes of the lumbar vertebrae medially.

C. The femoral nerve runs medial to psoas.

D. The obturator nerve passes over the anterior aspect of psoas.

E. The subcostal nerve, the iliohypogastric nerve, and the ilioinguinal nerve emerge from the lateral aspect of psoas major over quadratus lumborum.

True:	B E
False:	A C D

Figure 24 presents a diagram of the posterior abdominal wall. The three muscles that form the posterior boundary of the abdomen are psoas major, quadratus lumborum, and iliacus. The attachments of quadratus lumborum are as stated above. Psoas major, however, attaches to the transverse processes and intervening intervertebral discs of T12–L5. The gaps it leaves over the vertebral bodies allows for the exit of the spinal nerves. Iliacus arises from the inner surface of the ilium of the pelvis and attaches *via* the tendon of psoas into the lesser trochanter of the femur. Various important nerves are related to psoas major and these are shown below (note that the three nerves that pass to the anterior abdominal wall emerge from the lateral border of psoas).

Lateral border psoas

- Subcostal n. (T12)
- Iliohypogastric n. (L1)
- Ilioinguinal n. (L1)
- Femoral n. (L2–L4)

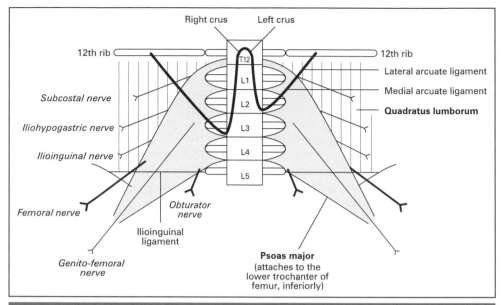

Right crus   Left crus

12th rib

T12
L1
L2
L3
L4
L5

Subcostal nerve

Iliohypogastric nerve

Ilioinguinal nerve

Femoral nerve

Ilioinguinal
ligament

Genito-femoral
nerve

Obturator
nerve

Psoas major
(attaches to the
lower trochanter of
femur, inferiorly)

12th rib
Lateral arcuate ligament
Medial arcuate ligament
Quadratus lumborum

Fig. 24 The diaphragm seen from the abdominal side, showing the main openings.

Over psoas

- Genito-femoral n. (L1–L2)

Medial to psoas

- Obturator n. (L2–L4)

12. The diaphragm (superior abdominal wall).

A. It originates from the lower six costal cartilages.

B. The arcuate ligaments are thickenings of the fascia of psoas and quadratus lumborum.

C. It has no attachment to the xiphoid.

D. It is pierced by the oesophagus at T10.

E. The left phrenic nerve passes through with the aorta.

True:	A B D
False:	C E

The diaphragm (*Figure 25*) is considered here as it forms the muscular superior abdominal wall. It arises from the lower six costal cartilages laterally, the xiphoid anteriorly, and the arcuate ligaments and crura posteriorly. The medial and lateral arcuate ligaments are fibrous thickenings of the fasciae of psoas and quadratus lumborum, respectively. The left crus arises from L1–L2; the right crus of the diaphragm arises from L1–L3 and passes up around the oesophagus. The diaphragm is pierced by the following structures:

- Right phrenic nerve with IVC at T8 (note: the left phrenic nerve pierces the diaphragm alone).

- Oesophagus with right vagus posteriorly and left anteriorly at T10.

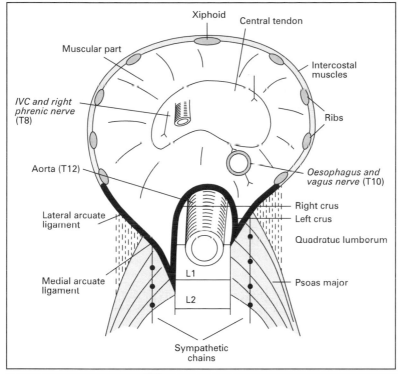

Fig. 25 Posterior abdominal wall. The diagram shows the two muscles (psoas major and quadratus lumborum) forming the posterior abdominal wall, and the thickening of fascia which form the right and left crura and the arcuate ligaments. The medial arcuate ligament is a thickening of the quadratus lumborum fascia. Also shown are the nerves of the posterior abdominal wall and their relation to psoas major.

- Aorta with thoracic duct at T12.
- Splanchnic nerves.
- Sympathetic chain behind medial arcuate ligaments.

13.   The peritoneum.

A.   The greater omentum consists of two layers of peritoneum.

B.   The lesser omentum connects the stomach and the liver.

C.   The origin of the mesentery of the small intestine (SI) runs obliquely across the posterior abdominal wall, from the upper right region to the left sacro-iliac joint.

D.   The stomach is a retroperitoneal organ.

E.   The pancreas is retroperitoneal.

True:	B E
False:	A C D

The peritoneum of the abdomen is derived from the same embryological structure as the pleura in the thorax. To understand the longitudinal folds of the peritoneum, it is useful to

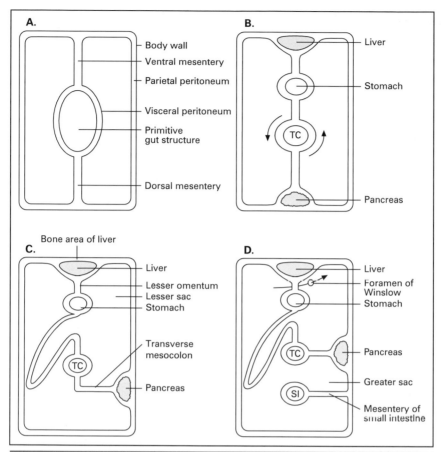

Fig. 26 A much simplified diagrammatic representation of the development of the abdominal peritoneum, which helps the student understand how the omenta and mesenteries are formed. Note the four layers of the greater omentum. SI = small intestine; TC = transverse colon.

compare the peritoneum with the pleura. The peritoneum has a visceral layer (adherent to the organs) and a parietal layer (adherent to the abdominal walls) in the same way as the pleura. However, whereas the visceral pleura fold in on the lung to form a single hilum to carry nerves and vessels to the lung, the peritoneum has two such folds, known as the dorsal and ventral mesentery, in the developing abdomen (*Figure 26A*). These two mesenteries meet and enclose part of the liver, the whole of the stomach and transverse colon (TC), but not the pancreas, which remains retroperitoneal. As the abdomen grows, the contents of the abdomen move and, as they do so, pull the mesenteries with them (*Figure 26B*). This results in a fold of double-layered visceral peritoneum between the stomach and TC. This adheres to form the quadruple-layered greater omentum below the TC (*Figure 26C*). The fold of peritoneum between the liver and the stomach is known as the lesser omentum. The space between the lesser omentum and the mesentery of the TC below, is known as the lesser sac. Only two details need to be added to this picture. First, there is a separate mesentery for the SI (*Figure 26D*) running obliquely from the left side of the body of L1 to the right sacro-iliac joint below. Second, due to the twisting of the developing gut, the lesser sac has an opening on its right side known as the epiploic foramen of Winslow (*see* Question 14).

14.   The lesser sac.

A.   Lies anterior to the stomach.

B.   Has the pancreas as an anterior relation.

C.   Has no connections with the main peritoneal cavity.

D.   The aorta and IVC lie anterior to the epiploic foramen of Winslow.

E.   The portal triad lies posterior to the epiploic foramen of Winslow.

All false.

The lesser sac lies behind the stomach and in front of the pancreas. It is a pouch that lies behind the lesser omentum. The right side of the sac opens into the main peritoneal cavity via the foramen of Winslow (epiploic foramen). The left wall is formed by the spleen. *Figure 27* shows the relations of the foramen of Winslow, and presents a cross-section through the abdomen, to outline the peritoneal lining.

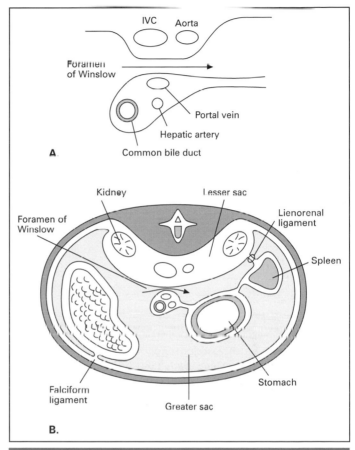

Fig. 27 Cross-sections, seen from above, of **A** the foramen of Winslow, and **B** the peritoneal cavity, in the upper abdomen. IVC = inferior vena cava.

UPPER ABDOMEN AND INTESTINES

15.   The stomach.

A.   The fundus bulges up above the cardia.

B.   The incisura marks the junction of the body with the antrum.

C.   The diaphragm is an anterior, superior and posterior relation of the stomach.

D.   The pyloric sphincter is formed by the thickening of the longtitudinal muscle layer.

E.   The lesser omentum is a double fold of peritoneum connecting the stomach to the liver.

True:	A B C E
False:	D

The cardia is the junction of the oesophagus and the stomach. Bulging up to the left is the gas-filled fundus, which can often be seen on a chest radiograph. The body of the stomach becomes the antrum at the incisura, the sharp notch on the lesser curvature. The incisura is a permanent feature and does not vary with peristalsis. The anterior relations of the stomach are the diaphragm, the left lobe of the liver and the abdominal wall. The diaphragm lies above the stomach, while behind the stomach lie the two layers of the lesser sac and then a host of important structures known collectively as the stomach bed. This consists of the left crus of the diaphragm, the left kidney and adrenal gland, the spleen, the pancreas, the transverse mesocolon, the splenic artery and, just to the right of the mid-line, the aorta with its coeliac axis. The pylorus is a thickening of the circular muscle; it can be palpated at dissection. The lesser omentum hangs down from the liver to the lesser curvature of the stomach. The greater omentum hangs down off the greater curvature of the stomach and attaches to the TC.

16.   The blood supply of the stomach.

A.   The right gastric artery gives off an important branch to the oesophagus.

B.   The lesser curvature of the stomach is supplied by the right and left gastric arteries.

C.   The short gastric arteries run in the gastro-splenic ligament.

D.   The right gastro-epiploic artery is a branch of the hepatic artery.

E.   The epiploic branches of the gastro-epiploic arteries supply the greater omentum and the TC to which it attaches.

True:	B C D
False:	A E

The stomach has a rich vascular supply (*Figure 28*) from the coeliac axis of the aorta at the level of T12. The lesser curvature is supplied by the right and left gastric arteries. The left gastric artery comes off the coeliac axis and gives a branch to the oesophagus.

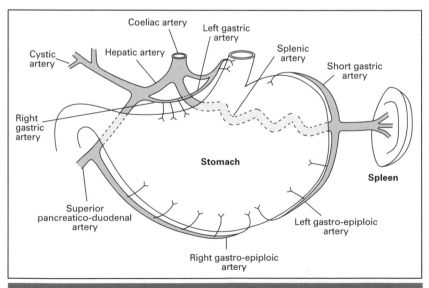

Fig. 28 The arterial supply to the stomach.

The corresponding vein forms an important portal-systemic anastomosis with the systemic drainage of the oesophagus and is important in oesophageal varices. The splenic artery runs across the pancreas to the spleen and supplies the stomach through the short gastric arteries, which run back to the upper part of the greater curvature in the gastro-splenic ligament and the left gastro-epiploic artery. The remainder of the greater curvature is supplied by the right gastro-epiploic artery, which comes off the gastroduodenal branch of the hepatic artery. Although the epiploic vessels supply the greater omentum right up to its junction with the TC, they do not supply the bowel itself.

17. The liver.

A.   The liver is entirely enclosed in peritoneum.

B.   The falciform ligament ascends from the umbilicus to reach the liver with the ligamentum teres in its free edge.

C.   The caudate lobe is anterior and lies between the gallbladder and the ligamentum teres.

D.   The quadrate lobe is functionally part of the left lobe of the liver.

E.   The surface marking of the liver reaches as high as the xiphisternal joint.

True:	B D
False:	A C E

The liver is enclosed in peritoneum, apart from a small bare area posteriorly. The falciform ligament ascends from the umbilicus with the ligamentum teres (remnant of the umbilical vein) in its free border. The ligamentum teres passes under the liver while the falciform ligament passes up over the liver and bifurcates. To the right it joins with the coronary ligament, and to the left it forms the left triangular ligament. The right triangular ligament is formed by the fusion of two layers of the coronary ligament. The quadrate and caudate lobes were once regarded as being anatomically part of the right lobe, but functional studies have shown them to be physiologically part of the left lobe. The quadrate lobe lies anteriorly between the gallbladder and ligamentum teres; the caudate is posterior between the IVC and ligamentum venosum. The surface marking of the liver is at the xiphisternal joint in the mid-line but reaches as high as the 5th rib on the right and 5th intercostal space on the left (approximately the nipple line).

18. The gallbladder.

A.   Stores up to 500 ml of bile.

B.   Has a surface marking at the tip of the 9th costal cartilage.

C.   lies in contact with the liver, the TC and the first part of the duodenum.

D.   Is supplied by the cystic artery via the right hepatic artery.

E.   Has its smooth muscle arranged in a spiral.

True:	B C D
False:	A E

The gallbladder has a capacity of around 50 ml. Its surface marking lies at the tip of the 9th costal cartilage where the transpyloric plane crosses the right costal margin. Its named artery is the cystic artery, which typically is a branch of the right hepatic artery. The gallbladder also receives a rich supply from the liver bed, however (this is why gangrene of the gallbladder is so rare). There is surprisingly little smooth muscle in the gallbladder. The 'spiral valve of Heisler' is formed by the arrangement of the mucous membrane. The neck of the gallbladder can dilate to form a diverticulum, known as Hartmann's pouch, where gallstones can impact.

19. The duodenum.

A. The duodenum has crypt-like glands opening into deep acini in the submucosa.

B. The first part of the duodenum is half peritoneal and half extra-peritoneal.

C. The duodenum is supplied by the pancreatico-duodenal arteries off the SMA.

D. The pancreatic duct and common bile duct open posteromedially half-way down the second part of the duodenum.

E. The duodeno-jejunal junction is well marked by a ligament which comes off the psoas fascia.

True:	A B D
False:	C E

The duodenum (*Figure 29*) is C-shaped, surrounding the head of the pancreas. It has distinctive deep crypts, known as Brunner's glands. The first 1 in. (2.5 cm) of the duodenum is covered with peritoneum before it becomes retroperitoneal. Half-way down the second part of the duodenum lies the duodenal papilla where the common bile duct and the main pancreatic duct (of Wirsung) open. This opening has an ampulla (of Vater) and is protected by a muscle sphincter (of Oddi). The secondary pancreatic duct (of Santorini) opens into the duodenum a little higher up. The superior pancreatico-duodenal artery is a branch of the gastroduodenal artery, which

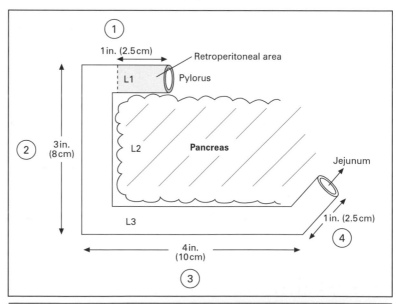

Fig. 29 Diagrammatic representation of the duodenum. The C-shaped duodenum has four parts (numerals 1–4 in circles) which loop around the pancreas from the pylorus of the stomach to the jejunum. The vertebral levels (L1, L2, and L3) of each part are indicated.

comes off the coeliac axis *via* the hepatic artery. The inferior pancreatico-duodenal artery is a branch of the SMA. The anastomosis half-way down the second part of the duodenum marks the meeting of foregut (supplied by the coeliac axis) and midgut (supplied by the SMA). The suspensory ligament of Treitz descends from the right crus of the diaphragm and, together with the inferior mesenteric vein, marks the end of the duodenum and start of the jejunum.

20.   The pancreas.

A.   The pancreas is a retroperitoneal structure.

B.   The neck of the gland lies within the transpyloric plane of Addison.

C.   The splenic artery runs along the top of the gland.

D.   The pancreatic duct opens into the duodenum at the Ampulla of Vater along with the common bile duct.

E.   The inferior mesenteric vessels travel from behind the pancreas into the root of the mesentery.

True:	A B C D
False:	E

The pancreas is a retroperitoneal organ, the secretions of which enter the duodenum to aid in the process of digestion. It consists of a head, neck, body and tail. The head lies within the C-shaped segment (1st–3rd parts of the duodenum). An extension of the head, the uncinate process, hooks posteriorly to the superior mesenteric vessels as they travel from behind the pancreas into the root of the mesentery. The neck bears attachment to the transverse mesocolon. The superior mesenteric vessels are embedded between the uncinate process and the neck of the pancreas. The splenic artery passes along the upper border of the body and the tail. Anteriorly, lie the lesser sac and stomach. Posteriorly, lie the IVC, aorta, common bile duct, superior mesenteric vessels, right and left renal veins, left crus of the diaphragm, left psoas muscle, left suprarenal gland, and the splenic vein. The splenic vein drains the inferior mesenteric vein that joins the superior mesenteric vein, finally forming the portal vein, behind the neck of the gland. The pancreatic duct of Wirsung runs from tail to head and is then joined by the common bile duct before it enters the 2nd part of the duodenum at the Ampulla of Vater. The uncinate process and lower aspect of the head of the pancreas are drained by the accessory pancreatic duct of Santorini. This often communicates with the main pancreatic duct and opens into the duodenum, approximately ¾ in. (2 cm) above it. For structures within the transpyloric plane of Addison (L1) *see* Question 3. The pancreas is supplied by the splenic artery, and the superior and inferior pancreatico-duodenal arteries.

21.   The spleen.

A.   The left lung and 9th, 10th, and 11th ribs lie posterior to the spleen.

B.   The spleen is fully encased in peritoneum.

C.   When the spleen is enlarged, a notch can be felt in its anterior border.

D. Accessory spleens are found in 10% of patients.

E. The spleen may be damaged in penetrating thoracic trauma.

All true.

The spleen is traditionally remembered as measuring $1 \times 3 \times 5$ in., weighing 7 ounces and lying on the 9th to 11th ribs. In these metric times, its size is perhaps best thought of as being that of a clenched fist. Its long axis lies along the 10th rib. The hilum lies in an angle between the stomach and the left kidney. The spleen is also in contact with the splenic flexure of the colon below, and is moulded into the diaphragm above and behind. It is fully encased in peritoneum, which, at the hilum, contacts the greater omentum to form two double layers. These run as ligaments: one to the stomach, carrying the short gastric and left gastro-epiploic arteries; and one to the left kidney, carrying splenic vessels. They are known as the gastro-splenic and lienorenal ligaments, respectively. Due to the formation of the spleen from multiple splenules, its anterior border is notched, and this can be felt when an enlarged spleen is palpated. Accessory splenules are found in 10% of subjects, often at the hilum or along the splenic vessels but they can be elsewhere in the abdomen. The spleen is at high risk in stab wounds to the left lower chest and, due to its thin, tense capsule, is the abdominal organ most frequently injured in blunt trauma.

22. The jejunum and ileum.

A. The mesentery of the SI comes off the anterior abdominal wall.

B. The plicae circulares are thicker in the jejunum than in the ileum.

C. Fat deposits are thicker in the mesentery of the jejunum than in that of the ileum.

D. The mesenteric vessels to the jejunum form fewer arcades than are formed by the vessels supplying the ileum.

E. Peyer's patches lie along the border of the mesentery and the lower ileum.

True:	B D
False:	A C E

The SI can be up to 33 feet (10 m) long; the average length is 24 feet (7.5 m). The mesentery originates from the posterior abdominal wall, commencing at the duodeno-jejunal flexure and passing down to the right sacro-iliac joint. The upper two-fifths of the small bowel is jejunum; the lower three-fifths is ileum. There is a gradual change in character between the two. Differences between the jejunum and ileum are shown diagrammatically in *Figure 30*. The jejunum is thicker walled, due to larger, thicker plicae circulares. In addition, the jejunum has a greater number of villi on its inner surface compared to the ileum. These differences give the two parts different textures when touched, with the jejunum being described as being like thick velvet and the ileum as being like thin paper. The jejunum has a wider diameter, less fat and a simpler blood supply than the ileum, which has complex vascular arcades. The jejunum tends to lie around the umbilicus, while the ileum coils into the hypogastrium and pelvis. The lower ileum has aggregations of lymphoid tissue known as Peyer's patches along the anti-mesenteric border.

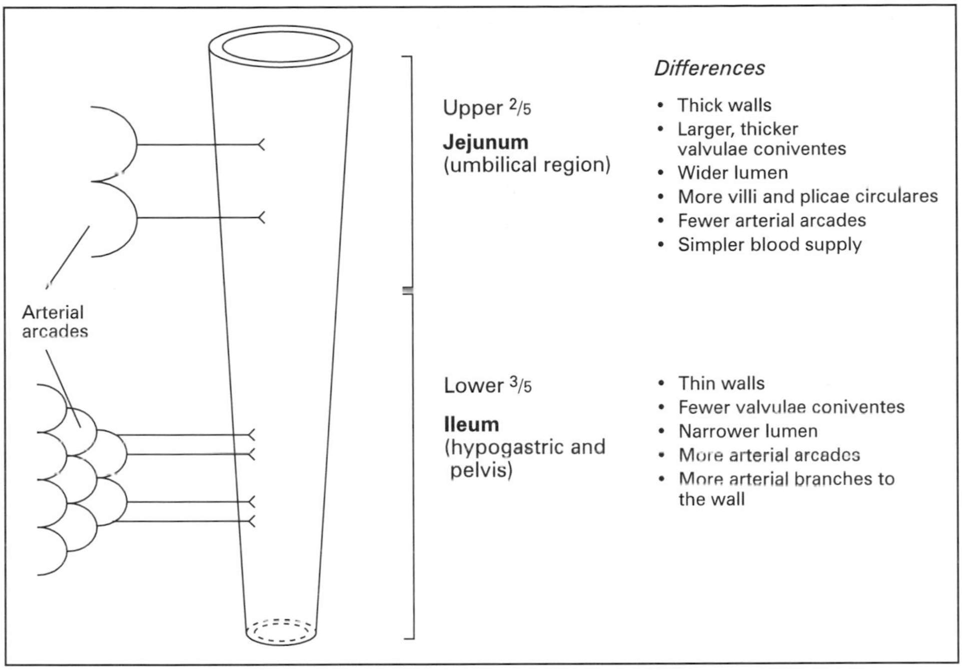

Arterial arcades
Upper 2/5
Jejunum
(umbilical region)
Differences
• Thick walls
• Larger, thicker valvulae coniventes
• Wider lumen
• More villi and plicae circulares
• Fewer arterial arcades
• Simpler blood supply
Lower 3/5
Ileum
(hypogastric and pelvis)
• Thin walls
• Fewer valvulae coniventes
• Narrower lumen
• More arterial arcades
• More arterial branches to the wall

Fig. 30 The main differences between the jejunum and the ileum.

23. The large bowel.

A. The colon has most of its longitudinal muscle gathered in three bands.

B. The descending colon has no mesentery.

C. The large bowel is supplied by both the inferior mesenteric and superior mesenteric arteries.

D. The sigmoid colon is the most frequent site of large bowel perforation.

E. The TC is extremely mobile.

All true.

The large bowel has its longitudinal muscle gathered into three flattened bands known as taeniae coli. These are visible on abdominal radiograph if the large bowel is distended. The ascending and descending colon usually have no mesentery (they do in at least 10% of subjects) but adhere to the posterior abdominal wall through pseudomesenteries, which form through a process known as zygosis. These pseudomesenteries do not carry vessels and can be cut through in the living quite safely. The TC is very mobile on its transverse mesocolon and can hang down into the pelvis. The SMA supplies large bowel up to two-thirds of the way along the TC, the remainder receives its blood from the inferior mesenteric artery. The sigmoid colon, being the most common site of diverticulitis, is the most likely part to perforate.

24. The appendix.

A. Arises from the postero-lateral surface of the caecum.

B. Has a surface marking half-way along a line between the ASIS and the symphysis pubis.

C. Receives its blood supply from a named branch of the ileocolic artery.

D. Is commonly between 2½ and 3½ in. (6 and 9 cm) in length.

E. Lies at the convergence of the taeniae coli of the caecum.

True:	C D E
False:	A B

The base of the appendix lies on the postero-medial surface of the caecum ¾ in. (2 cm) below the ileo-caecal valve. At operation, if the appendix is not immediately visible, the taeniae of the caecum can be followed until they converge at the base of the appendix to form a single longitudinal muscle layer. The length of the appendix can vary between 1 and 10 in. (2 and 25 cm) although it is most commonly between 2½ and 3½ in. (6 and 9 cm). The tip of the appendix is highly variable in position. It is most commonly retro-caecal or retro-colic at operation, although probably most often found in a retro-ileal position in the absence of disease. It can be found abutting the right kidney, against the duodenum or down in the pelvis. The appendicular artery is a branch of the ileocolic artery off the SMA. It runs down to the appendix in its mesentery, the mesoappendix. The appendix is often reached by a second mesentery known as the ileocolic fold, sometimes called the 'bloodless fold of Treves' (although it usually contains small vessels).

RETROPERITONEUM

25. The descending abdominal aorta.

A. The coeliac trunk is the first unpaired branch of the abdominal aorta.

B. The SMA lies at the level of L2.

C. There are only two paired visceral branches.

D. There are three terminal branches.

E. There are four paired lumbar arteries to the posterior abdominal wall.

True:	A D E
False:	B C

The aorta slips between the crura of the diaphragm at T12, and descends on the bodies of the lumbar vertebrae to L4, where it divides into the three terminal branches: left and right common iliac arteries, and the median sacral artery. It gives off three, anteriorly situated, unpaired visceral branches to supply the gut and its adnexae (liver, pancreas, and spleen): the coeliac trunk (T12); the SMA (L1); and the inferior mesenteric artery (L3). There are three paired visceral branches to the suprarenal glands, kidneys and gonads. There are five paired branches to the parietes: the inferior phrenic arteries (to diaphragm); and the four pairs of lumbar arteries to the posterior abdominal wall. The abdominal aorta and its branches are illustrated in *Figure 31*.

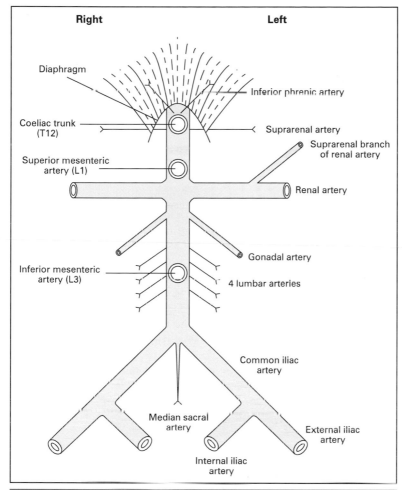

Fig. 31 The abdominal aorta and its branches. Note that there are three unpaired visceral branches anteriorly, three paired visceral branches, and five paired branches to the parietes.

26.   The abdominal inferior vena cava.

A.   It is formed by the confluence of the common iliac veins and median sacral vein at the level of L5.

B.   It runs under the right common iliac artery.

C.   The left renal vein runs into it over the aorta, inferior to the SMA.

D.   It receives three paired visceral tributaries (suprarenal, renal and gonadal veins) directly.

E.   It has three anteriorly placed unpaired visceral veins draining the gut and its adnexae.

True:	**A B C**
False:	**D E**

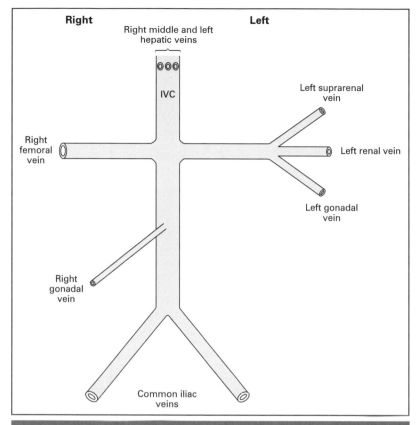

Fig. 32 The inferior vena cava (IVC) and its tributaries.

The left suprarenal and gonadal veins drain into the left renal vein. The gut drains *via* the portal system to the liver. The liver drains into the IVC *via* two or three hepatic veins. *See Figure 32.*

27. The adrenal glands.

A. They lie outwith the renal fascia.

B. They lie directly on the kidney and are surrounded by perirenal fat.

C. Their only blood supply comes directly from the aorta.

D. The left adrenal overlies the upper pole of the left kidney laterally.

E. The left adrenal vein drains directly to the IVC.

All false.

The right adrenal overlies the upper pole of the right kidney, whereas the left adrenal is more medially related and abuts onto the hilum of the left kidney. The adrenals lie within the renal fascia but are separated from the kidneys by the perirenal fascia. They receive a triple blood supply: the suprarenal arteries; the suprarenal branch of the renal artery; and the suprarenal branch of the inferior phrenic arteries. The glands drain by paired single veins, the right suprarenal directly to the IVC, and the left to the left renal vein.

28. The position and relations of the kidneys.

A. The hila lie at the level of L1.

B. The left kidney is slightly lower than the right.

C. The kidneys are directly covered by peritoneum anteriorly.

D. The head of the pancreas overlies the hilum of the right kidney.

E. Posteriorly the kidneys are separated from the lungs by the diaphragm.

True: **A**

False: **B C D E**

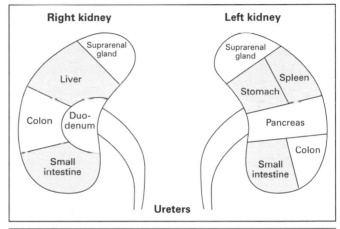

Fig. 33 Anterior relations of the kidneys. Shaded areas indicate an intervening layer of peritoneum between the kidneys and the overlying structure.

The anterior relations of the kidneys are shown in Figure 33 (note that, although entirely retroperitoneal, they are not entirely directly related to the peritoneum). Posteriorly they are separated by the diaphragm from the costodiaphragmatic recess and the 12th rib.

29. The blood supply of the kidneys.

A. The right renal artery usually overlies the IVC.

B. The renal vein lies anterior to the renal artery.

C. There are five segmental branches from each renal artery.

D. All the segmental branches pass anterior to the renal pelvis.

E. The lobar arteries are embedded within the substance of the kidney.

True: **B C**

False: **A D E**

The renal arteries arise from the abdominal aorta below the SMA and divide into five segmental arteries. The right renal artery usually passes behind the IVC, but there may be an aberrant artery passing anteriorly. The renal veins lie anterior to the renal pelvis. Therefore, the structures of the renal hilum (from anterior, running posteriorly) are as follows: renal vein; segmental arteries; pelvic ureter; and segmental artery (V/A/U/A). Of the five segmental arteries, four pass anterior to the renal pelvis and one posteriorly. The segmental arteries divide into lobar arteries (one for each pyramid), and the lobar into two or three interlobular arteries which enter the substance of the kidneys.

30. The ureters.

A. They run medial to psoas major.

B. They pass under the bifurcation of the common iliac arteries.

C. They are crossed by the gonadal vessels.

D. They receive their blood supply from paired ureteric arteries directly from the aorta.

E. The root of the mesentery of the SI overlies the right ureter at the sacro-iliac joint.

True:	C E
False:	A B D

The ureters are 10 in. (25 cm) long, and in the abdomen they are attached to the posterior aspect of the peritoneum. They run along the anterior surface of psoas major, which separates them from the tips of the transverse processes of the lumbar vertebrae behind. They enter the pelvis anterior to the sacro-iliac joint by crossing over the bifurcation of the common iliac arteries. Anteriorly, both ureters are crossed by the gonadal vessels. In addition, the right ureter is crossed by the right colic and ileocolic vessels, and the left ureter is crossed by the left colic vessels. The lower end of the mesentery of the SI overlies the right ureter at the sacro-iliac joint. The ureters receive their blood supply from the renal arteries, the gonadal arteries and the superior vesicular arteries.

3. Pelvis

TOPIC CHECK LIST

BOUNDARIES OF THE PELVIS

1. The bony pelvis.

A. The sacrum consists of five fused vertebral bodies.

B. In the erect position, the ASIS and the pubic symphysis lie in the same vertical plane.

C. The iliac crest lies at the level of L3.

D. The sacro-iliac joint is a fibrocartilaginous joint.

E. The posterior superior iliac spine (PSIS) lies at the level of S2.

True:	A B E
False:	C D

The pelvic girdle consists of two hip (innominate) bones, the sacrum and coccyx. The hip bone is a large, irregularly-shaped bone composed of three flat bones – the ilium, ischium and pubis – which are fused together in the adult at the acetabulum (fusion occurs between 15 and 25 years). The two hip bones articulate anteriorly at the pubic symphysis, which is a cartilaginous joint with an intervening disc of fibrocartilage. Posteriorly, the auricular surfaces of the two bones join by synovial plane joints to the auricular facets of the sacrum. The sacrum is a triangular bone derived from five fused vertebral bodies which form a central mass, the corresponding fused transverse process forming lateral masses. The sacral prominence is formed by the anterior border of the central mass. The sacral canal is formed by the fused vertebral arches. In the erect position, the ASIS and pubic symphysis lie in the same vertical plane. This can be demonstrated by placing a free pelvis against the wall. In this position it can be seen that the pubic symphysis and coccyx lie in the same horizontal plane. Important surface landmarks of bony pelvis and their vertebral levels are as follows:

- Iliac crest (L4)
- ASIS (S1)
- PSIS (S2)

2. The true and false pelvis.

A. The false pelvis lies above the iliopectineal line.

B. The outlet of the true pelvis is diamond shaped.

C. The sacrospinous and sacrotuberous ligaments form the lateral borders of the outlet of the true pelvis.

D. The pubic symphysis forms the anterior wall of the false pelvis.

E. The greater and lesser sciatic foramina are bounded by bone around their entire circumferences.

True:	A B C
False:	D E

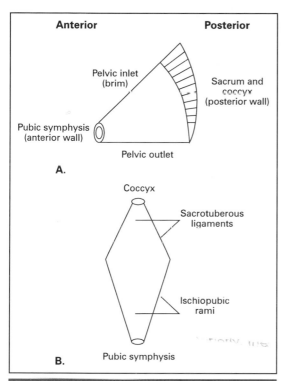

The pelvic brim is formed by the sacral prominence, iliopectineal line and symphysis pubis. The false pelvis lies above the pelvic brim (really the lower part of the abdominal cavity) and the true pelvis lies below. The true pelvis is, therefore, a short curved canal with a shallow anterior wall (pubic bodies and pubic symphysis) and a deeper posterior wall (sacrum and coccyx). The pelvic inlet corresponds to the pelvic brim. The pelvic outlet is bounded by the coccyx posteriorly, the ischial tuberosities laterally, and the pubic arch anteriorly. In addition, note the presence of two important ligaments: the sacrotuberous ligament and the sacrospinous ligament, which cross one another to convert the greater and lesser sciatic notches into the important greater and lesser sciatic foramina. The pelvic outlet is, therefore, diamond shaped with the boundaries shown in Figure 34

Fig. 34 A. Sagittal section of the pelvis, showing anterior and posterior boundaries. **B.** Boundaries of the diamond-shaped pelvic outlet, seen from above.

3. The female pelvis compared to the male pelvis.

A. The female pelvic inlet is more heart-shaped.

B. The female pelvis is longer in the cephalo-caudal direction.

C. The ischial tuberosities are more inverted in the female.

D. The pubic arch (subpubic angle) is smaller in the female.

E. The female pelvic outlet is more oval.

All false.

There are many differences between the male and female pelvis but the following are perhaps the most readily identifiable:

- The pelvic inlet is oval in female but heart shaped in the male; this is due to a bigger sacral promontory in the male.

- There is a wider, but shorter pelvis, in the female.

- In the female, the pelvic outlet is larger than in the male, with more everted ischial tuberosities.

- The pubic arch (subpubic angle) is greater in the female than in the male.

- The pelvic outlet in the female is more rounded than that of the male, which is more oval.

4. The walls of the pelvis, and the pelvic floor.

A. The piriformis muscle forms part of the posterior wall and passes through the greater sciatic foramen.

B. The obturator internus muscle forms part of the lateral wall and passes through the greater sciatic foramen.

C. There are no muscles on the anterior wall.

D. The sacral plexus lies deep to piriformis.

E. The muscles of the pelvic floor arise entirely from the bony pelvis.

True:	A C
False:	**B D E**

There are five walls to the pelvis (*Figure 35*): anterior, posterior, two lateral, and pelvic floor (pelvic diaphragm).

Anterior wall

• Pubic bone and pubic symphysis.

Posterior wall

• Sacrum and coccyx.

• Piriformis muscle: lateral mass of the sacrum, through the greater sciatic foramen, to the greater trochanter of the femur (lateral rotator of hip).

• Sacral plexus of nerves overlies piriformis.

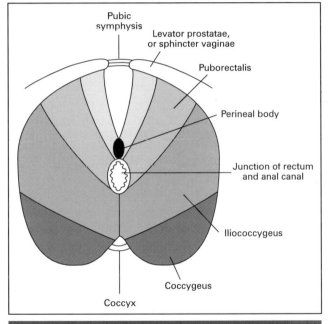

Fig. 35 The muscles of the pelvic floor.

Lateral wall

• Hip bone and ligaments.

• Obturator membrane and overlying obturator internus muscle: from hip bone and obturator membrane through the lesser sciatic foramen to greater trochanter of hip (lateral rotator of hip).

Pelvic floor (pelvic diaphragm)

• Levator ani muscle: arises from the body of the pubis and the fascia over obturator internus, and fibres swing inferomedially to several insertions which divide the muscle into several named groups of fibres (levator prostatae or sphincter vaginae, puborectalis and iliococcygeus).

• Coccygeus muscle: ischial spine to coccyx.

Note: The pelvic diaphragm splits the true pelvis into the main pelvic cavity above and the perineum below.

PELVIC VISCERA

5.   The contents of the male pelvis.

A.   The rectum lies directly behind the bladder.

B.   The ureters pass under the bifurcation of the common iliac artery at the pelvic brim.

C.   The prostate lies below the bladder, under the pelvic diaphragm.

D.   The ureters are crossed by the vasa deferentia prior to entering the bladder.

E.   The ureters enter the bladder anteriorly.

True:	A D
False:	**B C E**

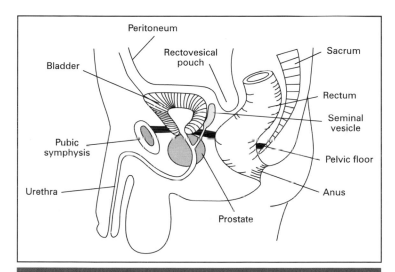

Fig. 36 Sagittal section of the male pelvis.

The following points about the arrangement of the male pelvis should be appreciated. The ureters enter the pelvic inlet at the bifurcation of the common iliac artery and run in front of the internal iliac artery (IIA) to the ischial spines, where they then turn medially to enter the bladder posteriorly. Just before entering the bladder they are crossed by the vasa deferentia (which carry sperm from the epididymis to the ejaculatory duct and urethra). The seminal vesicles (which produce secretion that is added to the seminal fluid to nourish the spermatozoa) lie inferior to the entry of the ureters into the bladder and medial to the ampullae of the vasa deferentia. The joining of each seminal vesicle and vas deferens gives rise to an ejaculatory duct. Each ejaculatory duct pierces the prostate gland to enter the urethra. The prostate (which produces alkaline secretion to neutralise the acidity of the vagina) is about 1¼ in. (3 cm) long, chestnut shaped, and lies below the bladder, separating it from the pelvic diaphragm. The rectum lies directly behind the bladder separated only by the recto-vesical space. *Figure 36* presents a sagittal section of the male pelvis.

6.   The contents of the female pelvis.

A.   The rectum lies directly behind the bladder.

B.   The ureters pass over the uterine arteries.

C.   The ovarian and round ligaments are the equivalent of the male gubernacula testes.

D.   The ligamentous supports of the uterus lie below the muscular pelvic diaphragm.

E.   The ovarian vessels pass up through the broad ligament of the uterus.

True:	C
False:	A B D E

A cross-section of the female pelvis is shown in *Figure 37*. The rectum and bladder in the female are separated by the vagina. Anterior to the uterus lies the vesico-uterine space, while posteriorly lies the recto-uterine space (Pouch of Douglas). The uterine arteries pass up inside the vertical fold of peritoneum that forms the broad ligament of the uterus. The uterine arteries pass over the top of the ureters and

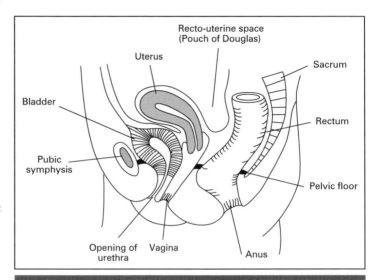

Fig. 37 Sagittal section of the female pelvis.

are highly convoluted to allow for expansion of the uterus during pregnancy. The ovarian vessels run down to the broad ligament from the infundibulo-pelvic ligament. There are three ligamentous supports to the uterus that lie above the pelvic diaphragm: the pubocervical ligament; the transverse cervical ligament; and the sacrocervical ligament.

7.   The prostate.

A.   Is about 4 cm × 3 cm × 2 cm.

B.   Lies below the urogenital diaphragm.

C.   Cannot be felt on rectal examination.

D.   Has an apex at the lower end.

E.   Has the ejaculatory ducts piercing the posterior surface below the bladder.

True:	A D E
False:	B C

The prostate produces 30% of seminal fluid, and lies below the bladder and above the urogenital diaphragm (levator ani). The ejaculatory ducts pass obliquely through the central zone of the gland to open into the urethra, half-way down the prostate. The peripheral zone surrounds the central zone from behind and below, accounting for 75% of glandular tissue. In between the openings of the ejaculatory ducts in the urethra is the prostatic utricle, a small recess representing the fused ends of the paramesonephric ducts (which forms the uterus in the female). The proximal urethra passes through the entire length of the prostate.

8. The urinary bladder.

A. The neck of the external sphincter is formed by the smooth muscle of the bladder.

B. SI and sigmoid colon lie on the superior surface of the bladder.

C. The trigone is a triangular area at the apex of the bladder.

D. Peritoneum entirely covers the bladder.

E. The external sphincter is under voluntary control.

True:	B E
False:	A C D

When empty, the bladder lies within the pelvic cavity, on the pubic symphysis and floor of the pelvis. It distends, separating the peritoneum from the anterior abdominal wall as far as the umbilicus, as it extends into the abdominal cavity. It has a smooth muscle wall called the detrusor muscle and is covered by transitional epithelium. The internal wall of the bladder has irregular folds, called trabeculae, and a smooth triangular area at the base, between the two ureteric orifices and the urethral orifice, called the trigone. Only the uppermost area of the bladder, between the ducti deferentia that lie on the bladder, is covered by peritoneum.

The internal sphincter is formed by the circular arrangement of the smooth muscle of the bladder wall at the neck of the bladder. The detrusor muscle and internal sphincter are under autonomic control and cannot be controlled voluntarily. Parasympathetic fibres cause contraction of the detrusor muscle and relaxation of the internal sphincter, thereby allowing micturition. Sympathetic fibres cause relaxation of the detrusor muscle and contraction of the internal sphincter. The external sphincter is under voluntary control. In the male, the external sphincter lies below the prostate.

The bladder receives its blood supply from the superior and inferior vesical arteries, branches of the internal iliac arteries.

9. The rectum.

A. Is lined by squamous epithelium.

B. Is supported by the levator ani muscle laterally.

C. Is entirely covered in peritoneum.

D. Begins at the level of the third sacral segment.

E. Has Denonvilliers' fascia as an anterior relation.

True:	B D E
False:	A C

The rectum is 5 in. (13 cm) in length, and commences at the third sacral segment, later becoming continuous with the anal canal. Anterior relations include: Denonvilliers' fascia; the bladder; and the prostate and seminal vesicles (in the male) and the vagina and uterus (in the female). Posteriorly, lie the sacrum, coccyx and the middle sacral artery, along with the rectal vessels and lymphatics. Peritoneum covers the upper two-thirds of the rectum anteriorly and laterally. In the middle third of the rectum, peritoneum covers the rectum only anteriorly. The peritoneum is then reflected upward from this point onto the bladder in the male, and vagina in the female, to form the Pouch of Douglas. This pouch contains small bowel and occasionally sigmoid colon, and represents the lowest part of the peritoneum in the abdomen. The blood supply to the rectum is from the superior rectal (primarily), middle, inferior and median sacral arteries. The veins follow the arteries, but anastomose freely with each other, so that the superior rectal vein drains to the portal system and the inferior to the systemic circulation. Lymphatic drainage is to the pararectal, preaortic and internal iliac nodes.

10. Structures palpable *via* a digital per rectum examination.

A. Coccyx

B. Prostate

C. Cervix

D. Seminal vesicles

E. Sacrum

True:	A B C E
False:	D

The structures that can be palpated through the anal canal, in either males or females, include: coccyx; sacrum; ischial spines; and the ano-rectal ring (shelf-like projection, which one's finger hooks around, separating the anal canal from the rectum). In the male, the prostate can be felt, but the seminal vesicles are not usually palpable. In females, one can feel the cervix, perineal body and occasionally the ovaries.

BLOOD SUPPLY AND NERVES OF THE PELVIS

11. The blood supply of the pelvis.

A. The gonadal arteries are branches of the IIA.

B. The superior rectal artery is a branch of the IIA.

C. The internal pudendal artery is a branch of the IIA.

D. The internal pudendal artery enters the perineum by piercing the levator ani muscle.

E. The inferior rectal artery is a direct branch of the IIA.

True:	C
False:	A B D E

The arterial supply to the pelvis is complex and confusing to most students. However, it can be more easily understood if one first considers which arteries actually enter the pelvis. Basically, there are two paired arteries and two unpaired arteries.

Two paired arteries enter the pelvis

- Internal iliac: from the bifurcation of the common iliac.
- Gonadal arteries: from the aorta high up in the abdomen.

Two unpaired arteries also enter the pelvis

- Median sacral: from the termination of the aorta into the common iliacs.
- Superior rectal: from the inferior mesenteric artery (lowest unpaired visceral branch of the abdominal aorta).

The IIA is the trunk of the main arterial tree to the pelvic viscera; it is shown diagrammatically in *Figure 38*. Note the following points:

- There is an anterior and posterior division to the IIA.
- There are branches to the lower limb which pass through the pelvic foramina:
  - obturator artery through the obturator canal;
  - gluteal arteries through the greater sciatic foramen.
- The internal pudendal artery, which supplies structures in the perineum, gets to the perineum by leaving the main pelvic cavity through the greater sciatic foramen and entering the perineum through the lesser sciatic foramen.
- The middle rectal artery is a direct branch of the internal iliac, but the inferior rectal artery is a branch of the internal pudendal.

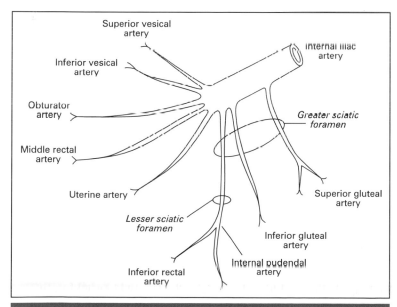

Fig. 38 Branches of the internal iliac artery.

12. The nerves of the pelvis.

A. The root values of the sacral plexus are L5–S4.

B. The internal iliac vessels lie behind the sacral plexus.

C. The pelvic sympathetic trunk lies lateral to the sacral foramina.

system and the inferior into the systemic, the anal canal forms an important communication between the two, i.e., an example of a porto-systemic anastomosis. Other important sites include oesophageal veins draining into the azygos vein (systemic) and left gastric vein (portal), and paraumbilical veins (portal) anastomosing with small epigastric veins of the anterior abdominal wall (systemic). It is possible that, if the pressure in the portal system increases, these tiny anastomotic veins engorge between both systems. In the anal region they are called haemorrhoids; in the oesophagus, varices; and on the abdominal wall, caput medusae. When in this state, they are likely to distend and even rupture, sometimes with fatal consequences (oesophageal varices). The wall of the anal canal constitutes a powerful sphincter mechanism. The internal is involuntary and is continuous with the circular muscle coat of the rectum. The external is voluntary and surrounds the internal sphincter. The upper end blends with the fibres of levator ani and in its lower component it traverses below the lower end of the internal sphincter.

EXTERNAL GENITALIA

16.   The male external genitalia.

A.   The penis is formed by three masses of erectile tissue.

B.   The urethra runs through the corpus cavernosum.

C.   The glans penis is formed from the corpus spongiosum.

D.   Vasodilatation of the penis is under sympathetic inervation.

E.   The penis contains no muscles.

True:	A C
False:	B D E

The penis is formed from three masses of erectile tissue arising from the ischiopubic rami and the perineal membrane. There are two corpora cavernosa and the corpus spongiosum, through which the urethra passes. All three masses of erectile tissue are surrounded by a fibrous sheath. Vasodilatation (erection) is under parasympathetic control, which reaches the penis *via* the pudendal nerve along with sensory fibres; ejaculation is under sympathetic control. There are four muscles at the base of the penis which assist in the production of an erection and in emptying the urethra at the end of micturition. The penis is surrounded by a layer of skin that, just behind the glans, is reflected on itself to form the retractable prepuce.

17.   The male and female external genitalia.

A.   The dartos muscle, in the scrotum, is derived from the IOM.

B.   The epididymis lies at the lower end of the spermatic cord, attached to the posterior border of the testes.

C.   Sensation to the scrotum is supplied by the ilioinguinal and genito-femoral nerves.

D.   In the female the clitoris lies anterior to the opening of the urethra.

E.   The labia minora lie medial to the labia majora.

True:	B C D E
False:	A

The scrotum is formed by a thin layer of skin, under which is a membranous superficial fascia which contains the dartos muscle. The function of this muscle is to draw the testes up nearer the body to increase testicular temperature in the cold. The cremaster muscle is derived from the IOM. The tunica vaginalis of parietal origin partially invaginates the testes. When fluid fills this space, a hydrocele is formed. The testes are covered by a thick fibrous layer, the tunica albuginea.

In the female the clitoris lies anterior to the urethral orifice which lies anterior to the vaginal opening. The urethra and vagina both open into the vestibule, which is surrounded by the labia minora. The two greater vestibular glands lie posteriorly on each side of the vaginal orifice. The clitoris is an erectile structure (equivalent to the male penis) that is enclosed in a fold of skin (the prepuce).

4. Upper Limb

TOPIC CHECK LIST

PECTORAL GIRDLE

1. The clavicle.

A. Most commonly fractures between the junction of middle and outer third.

B. Has no medullary cavity.

C. Ossifies late in fetal life.

D. Articulates with the coracoid process laterally, and with the manubrium of the sternum medially.

E. Articulates with the manubrium by a fibrous joint.

True:	A B
False:	C D E

The clavicle is the most commonly fractured bone in the body, and the medial fragment is classically elevated by the action of sternocleidonmastoid. Despite being a long bone, the clavicle is atypical in having no medullary cavity, reflecting its mostly membranous development. It is the first fetal bone to ossify. It articulates with the acromion of the scapula laterally (a plane synovial joint), its only connection to the coracoid process being through the coracoclavicular ligament. It is attached to the manubrium medially *via* a disc-containing synovial joint.

2. The joints and stability of the pectoral girdle.

A. The acromioclavicular joint has no disc.

B. The sternoclavicular joint involves the 1st costal cartilage.

C. The acromioclavicular joint is a fibrocartilaginous joint.

D. The coracoclavicular ligament provides no support to the clavicle.

E. The intraarticular disc of the sternoclavicular joint prevents medial movement of the clavicle.

True:	B E
False:	A C D

Both the sternoclavicular and acromioclavicular joints are synovial and both contain intraarticular discs. The disc of the sternoclavicular joint, together with the coracoclavicular ligament, provides vital support to the pectoral girdle by preventing medial movement of the clavicle. The sternoclavicular joint is a ball and socket joint and allows for rotation and circumduction of the clavicle. The acromioclavicular joint is a plane synovial joint and allows for elevation and anterior and posterior gliding of the acromion on the clavicle.

3. The scapula.

A. Has a superior and inferior angle overlying the 2nd and 7th ribs, respectively.

B. Is retracted by the action of the rhomboids.

C. Is rotated laterally by the actions of trapezius and serratus anterior.

D. Is separated from the trunk by serratus anterior alone.

E. Is attached to the trunk by pectoralis major.

True:	A B C
False:	D E

The palpable inferior angle of the scapula over the 7th rib is an important surface landmark. The scapula is attached to the trunk by six muscles: (anteriorly) pectoralis minor and serratus anterior; (posteriorly) trapezius, levator scapulae, and rhomboids major and minor. It is, however, separated from the trunk by serratus anterior and subscapularis. The middle fibres of trapezius assist the rhomboids in retracting the scapula, but the upper and lower fibres of trapezius assist the lower fibres of serratus anterior in lateral rotation of the scapula. The other movements, and the responsible muscles, are summarised below. All movements of the scapula reposition the orientation of the glenoid fossa, and increase the range of movement of the arm. Pectoralis major does not attach to the scapula but inserts directly into the humerus.

- Elevation: levator scapulae

- Depression: pectoralis minor

- Protraction: serratus anterior

- Retraction: rhomboids

4. The muscles connecting the pectoral girdle to the trunk.

A. Levator scapulae attaches to the spinous processes of C1–C4 vertebrae.

B. Serratus anterior attaches to the first eight ribs.

C. Pectoralis major has no attachment to the pectoral girdle.

D. Trapezius attaches to the skull, the ligamentum nuchae, and the supraspinous ligaments of the thoracic vertebrae.

E. The rhomboids attach to the medial border of the scapula below the level of the spine of the scapula.

True:	B C D E
False:	A

Levator scapulae attaches to the transverse processes of C1–C4 vertebrae and to the upper medial border of the scapula above the level of the spine of the scapula, whereas the rhomboids attach below. Serratus anterior attaches just lateral to the medial border of the scapula on its costal surface and to the upper eight ribs. Pectoralis major attaches to the medial part of the clavicle. Trapezius' attachment to the trunk runs from the superior nuchal line of the skull, down the ligamentum nuchae (the ligament overlying the cervical vertebrae), and the spinous processes and intervening supraspinous ligaments of all the thoracic vertebrae.

AXILLA

5. The boundaries of the axilla.

A. Pectoralis major forms part of the anterior wall.

B. Latissimus dorsi is part of the medial wall.

C. The apex is bounded by the 1st rib medially.

D. Coracobrachialis is situated laterally.

E. Subscapularis forms part of the posterior wall.

True:	A C D E
False:	B

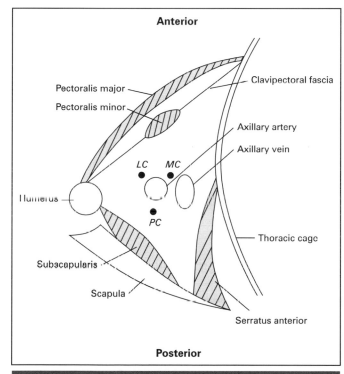

Fig. 39 Boundaries of the axilla and the relationship of the cords of the brachial plexus to the axillary artery. LC = lateral cord; MC = medial cord; PC = posterior cord.

The axilla is the name given to the fat-filled space which transmits all the nerves, vessels and lymphatics of the upper limb (i.e., the arm-pit). The axilla has the shape of a three-sided pyramid with anterior, posterior and medial walls. The walls of the axilla can easily be understood by referring to the diagram in *Figure 39*. Note how the two heads of biceps and coracobrachialis are situated laterally in the angle between the anterior and posterior walls. The apex of the axilla is situated superiorly, bounded by the 1st rib, clavicle and scapula. The floor of the axilla is formed by axillary fascia.

- Anterior wall: pectoralis major and minor (with clavipectoral fascia).
- Posterior wall: subscapularis, latissimus dorsi and teres major.
- Medial wall: serratus anterior and thoracic cage.

6. The clavipectoral fascia.

A. Forms the suspensory ligament of the axilla.

B. Encloses subclavius and pectoralis minor.

C. Encloses pectoralis major.

D. Is pierced by the cephalic vein.

E. Is pierced by the medial pectoral nerve.

True:	**A B D E**
False:	**C**

The clavipectoral fascia splits to enclose subclavius and pectoralis minor. Above pectoralis minor, the clavipectoral fascia stretches between the coracoid processes and the 1st and 2nd costal cartilages, and is known as the costocoracoid membrane. Below pectoralis minor, the clavipectoral fascia stretches down to the axillary fascia, which it supports, and is sometimes called the suspensory ligament of the axilla. The clavipectoral fascia is pierced by the following structures.

• Cephalic vein.

• Acromiothoracic artery.

• Lateral pectoral nerve and medial pectoral nerves.

• Lymph vessels from the infraclavicular node.

Note: The medial pectoral nerve pierces pectoralis minor also.

7. The quadrangular and triangular spaces.

A. Are part of the posterior axillary wall.

B. Are bounded by subscapularis superiorly, and teres major inferiorly.

C. Are separated by the short head of triceps.

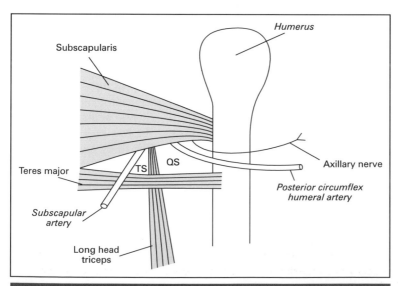

Fig. 40 The muscular boundaries of the QS and the TS, and the structures which pass through the two. QS = quadrangular space; TS = triangular space.

D. The quadrangular space (QS) transmits the radial nerve.

E. The triangular space (TS) transmits the suprascapular artery.

True:	A B
False:	C D E

There is a horizontal triangular gap between subscapularis, teres major and the humerus, which is divided by the long head of triceps running posteriorly into a lateral QS and medial TS (shown in *Figure 10*). The QS is particularly important because it transmits the axillary nerve and posterior circumflex humeral artery. The TS transmits the subscapular artery. Note that teres major defines the lower border of the axilla because the posterior wall extends further inferiorly than the anterior wall.

8. The contents of the axilla.

A. The axillary artery is medial to the axillary vein.

B. The axilla contains the divisions of the brachial plexus.

C. There are two venae commitantes running with the axillary artery.

D. The axillary artery is a branch of the subclavian artery.

E. There is little fat in the axilla.

All false.

The axilla contains the axillary artery and vein, both of which are continuous with the subclavian and brachial vessels as they pass in and out of the axilla. The three cords of the brachial plexus are named according to their relationship to the axillary artery. The axillary vessels are considered in more detail in the section on blood supply to the upper limb.

9. The lymph nodes in the axilla.

A. There are over 100 nodes in the axilla.

B. The nodes can be classified surgically into three groups.

C. The lateral group receives lymph from the upper limb.

D. The central group is the final common pathway.

E. The apical group receives lymph from the supraclavicular nodes.

True:	B C
False:	A D E

Whilst it is not essential to know the exact number of nodes in the axilla, it should be appreciated that they number in the fifties rather than the thousands. They are arranged in five groups which can easily be understood and remembered by again considering the axilla as a pyramid. There is one group for the anterior walls and one group for the posterior walls of the pyramid, and a lateral group near the axillary vein. The sites of these three groups and the areas they drain are listed in the following sections.

Anterior (pectoral) group

- Situated along the border of pectoralis major.
- Drain front of chest (including 75% of breast) and abdomen.

Posterior (subscapular) group

- Situated anterior to subscapularis.
- Drain back from neck down to iliac crest.

Lateral group (venous) group

- Situated in lateral part of axilla along (and mostly medial to) the axillary vein (therefore obeying the general rule that lymphatics follow a venous path).
- Drain the whole of the upper limb.

The remaining two groups lie at the bottom and the top of the pyramid. The central group lie on the floor and are so named because they are situated in the centre of the floor rather than the centre of the pyramid. The apical (infraclavicular) group are aptly named because they lie in the apex of the axilla near the axillary vessels (occasionally there are one or two nodes in the deltopectoral groove). Both groups receive lymph from the other three axillary groups of nodes (in addition, the apical nodes may receive some lymph vessels running with the cephalic vein). However, the only exit for lymph from the axilla is through apical nodes to the subclavian trunk. The central nodes must, therefore, drain to the apical nodes. The lymph nodes in the axilla are sometimes classified surgically into three groups according to their relationship to pectoralis minor: group I below; group II behind; and group III above.

SHOULDER JOINT AND ROTATOR CUFF

10.   The structure of the shoulder joint.

A.   The labrum glenoidale is a fibrous ring around the joint capsule.

B.   Osteitis of the upper end of the humeral diaphysis may enter the joint capsule by direct spread.

C.   The head of the humerus forms three-fourths of a sphere.

D.   The subacromial bursa lies below the tendon of supraspinatus.

E.   The subscapular bursa usually communicates with the synovial cavity of the joint.

True:	B E
False:	A C D

The shoulder joint is a highly mobile but unstable joint. The labrum glenoidale is a cartilaginous intracapsular ring, which helps deepen the otherwise shallow glenoid fossa. The joint capsule itself is very lax and extends down onto the diaphysis of the medial aspect of the humerus, thus allowing for direct intraarticular spread of an osteitis. There are two large bursae associated with the shoulder joint. The subacromial bursa lies between the acromion and the tendon of supraspinatus, and when inflamed can be very painful (bursitis). The subscapularis bursa lies between subscapularis and the fibrous capsule of the joint, and usually communicates with the synovial cavity.

11. The stability of the shoulder joint.

A. The shoulder joint is strengthened primarily by its capsule.

B. The weakest position of the shoulder joint is in the adducted position.

C. The glenohumeral ligaments are vital supports.

D. The coracohumeral ligament prevents posterior dislocation.

E. The rotator cuff gives support to the inferior part of the joint.

All false.

The strength of the joint is determined by the shape of the bones, by the cartilage and ligaments, and by the rotator cuff muscles. The ball of the joint – the head of the humerus – forms one-third of a sphere, and inserts into the shallow socket of the glenoid cavity, thereby allowing for mobility but not providing stability. The glenoid labrum, a ring of fibrocartilage, encircles the glenoid cavity, making it deeper. The coracohumeral ligament, a thickening of the joint capsule which extends from the coracoid process to the

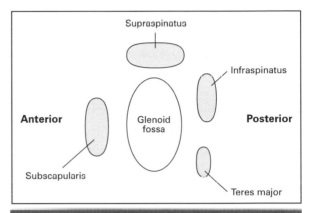

Fig. 41 Glenoid fossa seen from the side, showing how the rotator cuff muscles (see in cross-section) protect the superior, anterior and posterior aspects, but leave the inferior aspect unsupported.

anatomical neck of the humerus, prevents inferior dislocation of the adducted humerus. This ligament is tight only when the humerus is adducted and provides little stability in the abducted position. The coracoacromial ligament extends between the coracoid process and the acromion, and prevents superior displacement of the adducted humerus. Apart from the coracohumeral ligament, the rest of the joint capsule provides no strength (including the three glenohumeral ligaments). The muscles of the rotator cuff act as a muscular support to the shoulder joint: they surround the joint anteriorly (subscapularis), posteriorly (infraspinatus and teres minor), and superiorly (supraspinatus). The tendon of supraspinatus is fused to the underlying fibrous capsule. *Figure 41* shows that the rotator cuff does not strengthen the joint inferiorly. Supraspinatus, infraspinatus, and teres major sit (S.I.T.) on the facets of the greater tubercle of the humerus from above down. Subscapularis attaches to the lesser tuberosity.

12. Dislocation of the humerus.

A. Is usually posterior.

B. Usually occurs when the humerus is forcibly flexed.

C. May result in damage to the axillary nerve.

D.   Anterior dislocation is best corrected by Kocher's manoeuvre.

E.   Anterior dislocation results in medial displacement of the humerus.

True:	C D E
False:	A B

From the description given in Question 11, it can be seen that the inferior aspect of the shoulder joint is rather unprotected, and the humerus is most commonly dislocated into the infraglenoid region as a result of violent abduction. The strong adductors pull the humerus medially so that the acromion process is the most lateral bony prominence, as opposed to the greater tuberosity of the humerus. The QS lies immediately below the capsule of the shoulder joint, and the transmited axillary nerve and posterior circumflex humeral artery may be damaged. The axillary nerve supplies the deltoid muscle and teres minor and also skin over the so-called 'badge' area of the arm (over the lower fibres of deltoid). It is loss of sensation that indicates axillary nerve damage, as it will not be possible to test muscular function in a dislocated shoulder. Kocher's manoeuvre (traction on an externally rotated humerus followed by internal rotation) is the most commonly used method of reducing anterior dislocation.

13.   Movements of the shoulder joint.

A.   Supraspinatus is the main abductor.

B.   Pectoralis major adducts and medially rotates the humerus.

C.   Teres major is a lateral rotator and teres minor a medial rotator of the humerus.

D.   Deltoid is a flexor and extensor of the humerus.

E.   Pectoralis minor is a weak flexor.

True:	B D
False:	A C E

Supraspinatus is a very weak abductor of the humerus and after initiating abduction its main function may be in maintaining the stability of the humeral head in the glenoid during powerful abduction by deltoid. Deltoid has anterior, middle and posterior fibres: the anterior fibres assist humeral flexion; the posterior fibres assist in humeral extension. Teres major and teres minor both have origins on the posterior aspect of the scapula but their tendons insert, respectively, into the anterior and posterior aspects of the humerus. Teres major is, therefore, a medial rotator, while teres minor is a lateral rotator of the humerus. Pectoralis minor has no attachment to the humerus. Muscles acting on the humerus at the shoulder are summarised below.

Abduction

* Supraspinatus
* Deltoid

Adduction

* Pectoralis major
* Latissimus dorsi
* Teres major

Flexion

- Biceps
- Pectoralis major
- Deltoid – anterior fibres
- Coracobrachialis

Extension

- Triceps (long head)
- Teres major
- Deltoid (posterior fibres)

14. The surgical anatomy of the shoulder joint.

A. The coracoid process is an important landmark at the lower end of the deltopectoral groove.

B. The plane of cleavage between the infraspinatus and teres minor is a true internervous plane between the suprascapular nerve and the subscapular nerve.

C. There is no true internervous plane in a lateral approach to the shoulder.

D. The axillary artery is at risk in a lateral approach to the shoulder.

E. In the anterior approach to the shoulder the traction on coracobrachialis may damage the median nerve.

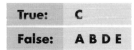

True: C

False: A B D E

The coracoid process protrudes anterolaterally from the scapula, and is important surgically because of its attachments and because it is also a landmark for the upper end of the deltopectoral groove. The coracoid attaches the coracoacromial and coracoclavicular ligaments and the tendons of the short head of biceps, coracobrachialis and pectoralis minor. There is no true internervous plane in the lateral approach to the shoulder as the fibres of deltoid are split longitudinally. Indeed, the axillary nerve, which supplies deltoid, is at risk in a lateral approach if the lateral incision is extended too far inferiorly. In a posterior approach there is a true internervous plane between the fibres of infraspinatus (suprascapular nerve) and teres minor (axillary nerve). In an anterior approach there is a true internervous plane between the fibres of supraspinatus (suprascapular nerve) and subscapularis (subscapular nerve). The following points regarding the course of the nerves around the shoulder are important to keep in mind when operating around the shoulder

- The axillary nerve passes through the QS (subscapularis and teres minor superiorly, surgical neck of humerus laterally, long head of triceps medially, teres major inferiorly) and is susceptible to damage here due to surgery, fractures or dislocations.

- The radial nerve passes through the triangular interval (teres major superiorly, long head of triceps medially, humerus laterally). The TS (subscapularis and teres minor superiorly, teres major inferiorly, long head of triceps laterally) conveys the circumflex humeral vessels.

- The musculocutaneous nerve passes through coracobrachialis and may be damaged through excessive traction on this muscle in the anterior approach.
- The suprascapular nerve is at risk if the supraspinatus muscle is mobilised too far medially.

HUMERUS AND COMPARTMENTS OF THE ARM

15. The relations and attachments of the humerus.

A. The axillary nerve passes around the anatomical neck.

B. The radial nerve crosses the anterior aspect of the midshaft at the mid-point.

C. The intertubercular groove contains the short head of biceps brachialis.

D. The ulnar nerve passes behind the medial epicondyle.

E. All three heads of triceps attach to the humeral shaft.

True:	D
False:	A B C E

The axillary nerve passes behind the surgical neck of the humerus where it is frequently damaged in humeral dislocation or surgical neck fractures. The radial nerve passes in the spiral groove on the posterior aspect of the humeral midshaft between the medial and lateral heads of triceps (the long head of triceps attaches to the infraglenoid tubercle of the scapula). The long head of biceps passes from the supraglenoid tubercle of the scapula and passes in the intertubercular groove between the greater and lesser tuberosities of the humerus.

16. The fascial compartments of the upper arm.

A. Coracobrachialis is contained within the anterior compartment.

B. All the main nerves of the upper limb pass through the anterior compartment, with the exception of the axillary nerve.

C. Both the cephalic and basilic veins pass through the anterior compartment.

D. The brachial artery runs within the posterior compartment.

E. The profunda brachii artery is the only artery passing through the posterior compartment.

True:	A B
False:	C D E

The humerus has a supracondylar ridge on both its medial and lateral aspects. From each ridge, a fascial septum extends to attach to the sheet of deep fascia that encloses the muscles of the upper arm. With the centrally placed humerus, these two septae divide the upper arm into the anterior and posterior fascial compartments. The triceps is the only muscle contained in the posterior compartment. Biceps, brachialis and coracobrachialis are contained within the anterior compartment. The musculocutaneous nerve runs within the anterior compartment, and supplies the muscles contained therein. The median and ulnar nerves also run in the anterior compartment. The radial nerve, which supplies triceps, passes for the most part through the posterior compartment, but traverses the lower part of the anterior compartment before entering the forearm. The brachial artery runs in the anterior compartment on the medial side of the upper arm. The profunda brachii and the ulnar collateral arteries run within the posterior compartment. Whilst the basilic vein enters the anterior compartment, the cephalic vein does not pass through either compartment but lies within the superficial fascia.

ELBOW JOINT AND ANTECUBITAL FOSSA

17. The elbow joint.

A. Flexion occurs at the humero-ulnar joint only.

B. The capitulum articulates with the ulnar.

C. The elbow joint has strong anterior and posterior ligaments.

D. The annular ligament encircles the capitulum.

E. Triceps extends the joint.

True:	E
False:	A B C D

The elbow joint is a single synovial joint with three articulations within the same capsule: the humero-ulnar joint between the trochlear of the humerus and the trochlear notch of the ulna (a hinge joint); the humeroradial joint between the capitulum of the humerus and the head of the radius (a ball-and-socket joint); and the proximal radioulnar joint between the radial head and the ulna (a pivot joint). The joint is reinforced by two collateral ligaments (medial and lateral) and an annular ligament around the radial head. Flexion and extension occurs at the humero-ulnar and humeroradial joints. Triceps attaches to the olecranon of the ulnar and extends the elbow, and is supplied by the radial nerve. Biceps (inserts into the radius) and brachialis (inserts into the ulnar) are the most powerful flexors of the elbow joint, and are both supplied by the musculocutaneous nerve. Pronation and supination take place at the proximal radioulnar joint with associated movements of the distal radioulnar joint. Pronation is brought about by pronator teres and pronator quadratus, both of which stretch between the radius and ulna on the anterior aspect of the forearm. Supination is brought about by supinator and by biceps. Biceps inserts into the medial aspect of the radius and so it is, in fact, the most powerful supinator – try opening a bottle of wine with a corkscrew and feel your biceps contract.

18. The surgical anatomy of the elbow.

A. The 'mobile wad of three' refers to brachoradialis, extensor carpi radialis longus and radialis brevis.

B. The posterior interosseous nerve is at risk during surgical approaches to the proximal ulna.

C. Posteriorly, the proximal ulna is crossed by the ulnar nerve.

D. In flexion the lateral and medial epicondyles and the proximal tip of the olecranon are in line.

E. Aspiration of the elbow is best performed anteriorly.

True:	A
False:	B C D E

The 'mobile wad of three' muscles all arise from the lateral supracondylar ridge and lateral epicondyle of the humerus. The posterior interosseous nerve passes through the supinator muscle near the neck of the radius to enter the posterior compartment of the forearm. It is vulnerable to damage, therefore, in any dissection near the proximal third of the radius. The ulnar nerve is obviously at risk in a medial approach to the elbow. However, there are no neural structures that cross the posterior aspect of the ulna. It is important to appreciate that the bony points of the elbow change position as the elbow is moved. In flexion the epicondyles and the tip of the olecranon form a triangle but are aligned when the elbow is in extension. Aspiration of the elbow is best done posteriorly well away from the structures of the antecubital fossa.

19.   The cubital fossa.

A.   Brachioradialis forms the lateral border.

B.   Pronator teres forms the medial border.

C.   Supinator forms the inferior border.

D.   The bicipital aponeurosis forms the roof of the fossa.

E.   The cubital fossa contains the median nerve.

True:	A B D E
False:	C

The cubital fossa is a triangular depression in front of the elbow joint. Brachioradialis and pronator teres form the lateral and medial borders, respectively, and the base of the triangle is an imaginary line drawn between the two epicondyles of the humerus. The bicipital aponeurosis overlies the structures within the fossa, which are (from lateral to medial) the tendon of biceps, the brachial artery and the median nerve (remembered by the TAN). The bicipital aponeurosis separates the artery from the median cubital vein, which crosses it superficially.

FOREARM

20.   The flexor (anterior) compartment of the forearm.

A.   Only flexor carpi ulnaris (FCU) is supplied by the ulnar nerve.

B.   The common flexor origin is the lateral epicondyle of the humerus.

C.   The median nerve runs deep to flexor digitorum superficialis (FDS).

D.   Palmaris longus is present in approximately 90% of individuals.

E.   Flexor pollicis longus is a superficial muscle.

True:	C D
False:	A B E

The common flexor origin is the medial epicondyle of the humerus. The muscles of the flexor compartment are divided into three groups: superficial; intermediate; and deep. The muscles in each group are listed below. All these muscles are supplied by the median nerve except for FCU and the ulnar (medial) half of flexor digitorum profundus. The median nerve lies immediately under FDS.

Superficial group

- Pronator teres
- Flexor carpi radialis
- Palmaris longus
- FCU

Intermediate group

- FDS

Deep group

- Flexor digitorum profundus
- Flexor pollicis longus

---

21. The extensor (posterior) compartment of the forearm.

A. Anconeus lies deep to extensor pollicis brevis.

B. Extensor carpi radialis longus is not part of the posterior compartment.

C. Abductor pollicis longus arises from the common extensor origin.

D. Extensor carpi ulnaris crosses above the extensor retinaculum.

E. All muscles of the posterior compartment of the forearm are supplied by the radial nerve.

True:	B E
False:	A C D

The muscles of the posterior compartment of the forearm can be split into a superficial and deep group (*see* list below). The superficial muscles arise from the common extensor origin (lateral humeral epicondyle). Both groups are supplied by the radial nerve, and all pass under the extensor retinaculum.

Superficial group

- Extensor carpi radialis brevis
- Extensor digitorum
- Extensor digiti minimi
- Extensor carpi ulnaris
- Anconeus

Deep group

- Supinator
- Abductor pollicis longus
- Extensor pollicis brevis
- Extensor pollicis longus
- Extensor indicis

Extensor carpi radialis longus and brachioradialis are the two muscles contained in the lateral compartment of the forearm. They are also supplied by the radial nerve.

WRIST AND HAND

The bones of the hand and wrist.

A. The carpal bones are connected by secondary cartilaginous joints.

B. The capitate is the largest carpal bone.

C. The pisiform is the last carpal bone to ossify, at about 12 months of age.

D. The first metacarpal articulates with the trapezium.

E. The hamate articulates with the radius.

True:	B C D
False:	A E

The skeleton of the hand consists of the eight carpal bones of the wrist, five metacarpals, and the 14 phalanges (three for each finger and two for the thumb). The carpal bones sit in two rows: a proximal row of three (triquetral, lunate, scaphoid) and a distal row of four (hamate, capitate, trapezoid, and trapezium). The pisiform overlies the triquetral and is a sesamoid bone (it lies in the tendon of FCU). The capitate is the largest carpal bone and is the first to ossify, at approximately 1 month of age. The chronology of the carpal ossification follows a spiral pattern, with the last to ossify being the pisiform (at 12 months). The hamate articulates with the ulnar only when the wrist is abducted to the ulnar side.

23. **The surgical anatomy of the wrist.**

A. The radial artery is at risk when inserting a K-wire into the radial styloid.

B. The anatomical snuff-box is bounded by the tendons of abductor pollicis longus anteriorly, and extensor pollicis brevis and extensor pollicis longus posteriorly.

C. The motor branch of the median nerve is best protected by making fairly laterally placed incisions in a volar approach to the wrist.

D. The median nerve lies medial to palmaris longus.

E. The tendons of FDS lie superior to palmaris longus.

True:	A B
False:	C D E

The wrist is a common site for operation due to the high incidence of distal radius fractures and carpal tunnel syndromes. K-wires are a fashionable method of stabilising distal radius fractures. Commonly, a K-wire is inserted into the radial styloid and directed proximally to help fix a distal bony fragment. The point of the skin incision is just distal to the radial styloid in the anatomical snuff-box, which is the small depression on the lateral aspect of the wrist formed by the tendons of abductor pollicis longus anteriorly, and of extensor pollicis brevis and extensor pollicis longus posteriorly. The following structures are at risk in the anatomical snuff-box: radial artery, the cephalic vein and the superficial radial nerve. A volar approach to the wrist is used in a carpal tunnel decompression. Usually, a 5 cm longitudinal incision is made from just distal to the flexor crease of the wrist running medial to the thenar skin crease towards the space between the ring and middle fingers. This keeps the knife on the ulnar side of the motor branch of the median nerve.

The palmar fat is cut until transverse fibres of the flexor retinaculum are identified. The flexor retinaculum is incised to release the pressure on the median nerve. In any volar approach to the wrist it is important to remember the relations of structures passing over the wrist joint. From lateral to medial these are: radial artery; flexor carpi radialis tendon; median nerve; palmaris longus tendon (flexor digitorum tendons lie underneath); ulnar artery; ulnar nerve; and FCU tendon.

24. The small muscles of the hand.

A.   There are eight interossei.

B.   The dorsal interossei abduct the fingers.

C.   The lumbricals extend the metacarpophalangeal (MCP) joints.

D.   All lumbricals are supplied by the ulnar nerve.

E.   The interossei arise from the metacarpals.

True:	B E
False:	A C D

There are seven interossei: three palmar interossei adduct the fingers and four dorsal interossei abduct the fingers. The ulnar nerve supplies all the interossei and the lateral two lumbricals. Because the interossei and lumbricals attach to the dorsal digital expansions, they extend the proximal interphalangeal (PIP) joints but flex the MCP joints.

25. The carpal tunnel and spaces of the hand.

A.   Flexor retinaculum extends from the hook of the hamate to the tubercle of the scaphoid.

B.   FCU passes through the carpal tunnel.

C.   FDS and flexor digitorum longus (FDL) pass through the carpal tunnel with the median nerve.

D.   The carpal bursa and radial bursa communicate in 50% of cases.

E.   Flexor pollicis longus is in the mid palmar space.

True:	A C D
False:	B E

There are four types of anatomical space in the wrist and hand: the fibrous carpal tunnel of the wrist; synovial spaces around tendons; pulp spaces of the fingers; and palmar fascial spaces. They are of particular significance as they help us understand the spread of infection in the hand. Also, at the wrist, the flexor retinaculum runs transversely over underlying tendons to form a fibrous tunnel known as the carpal tunnel. The flexor retinaculum extends from the piriform and the hook of the hamate medially to the tubercle of the scaphoid and trapezium laterally. The carpal tunnel contains all the long flexors of the fingers and thumb (flexor digitorum profundus, FDL and flexor pollicis longus) and the median nerve. Around the flexor tendons in the hand, there are synovial sheaths which allow the tendons to slide easily during muscular action. There are individual digital synovial sheaths for each of the fingers. In addition, there are synovial sheaths around the tendons of the long flexors in the carpal tunnel, which have fused to become two bursae known as the ulnar bursa and the radial bursa. The ulnar bursa contains all the long flexors of the fingers and communicates with the digital synovial sheath of

the little finger. The radial bursa
extends around flexor pollicis longus
to the digital synovial sheath of the
thumb. The radial and ulnar bursae of
the wrist are fused in 50% of cases
and this explains how infection in the
thumb may spread to the little finger.
The synovial spaces are shown in
Figure 42. The pulp spaces of the
fingertips consist of subcutaneous fat
broken up and packed between
fibrous septae extending between the
skin and periosteum. These spaces
are clinically significant because they
are tightly packed and infection,
although extremely painful, is usually
localised. The palmar spaces are
potential spaces between the fasciae
of the hand and are filled with
connective tissue. The fasciae
involved are the palmar aponeurosis,
septae diving dorsally from the
aponeurosis, and the fasciae of the
muscles. The two main spaces are
the midpalmar space and the thenar
space. Infection in these two
compartments tends to spread
dorsally.

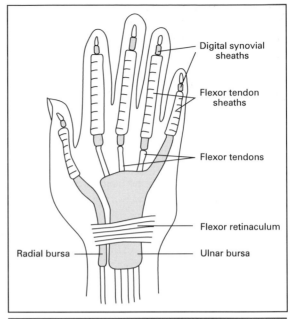

Fig. 42 The flexor tendon sheaths and the synovial tendon
sheaths of the left hand. Note how the ulnar bursa
communicates with the digital synovial sheath of the little finger,
and how that of the radial bursa communicates with the digital
synovial sheath of the thumb. The digital sheaths of the index,
middle and ring fingers do not communicate with ulnar or
radial bursae. In approximately 50% of the population, the
ulnar and radial bursae communicate; infection in the thumb
may therefore spread to the little finger.

---

26.   The thenar eminence.

A.   All muscles of the thenar eminence arise from the flexor retinaculum.

B.   Opponens pollicis (OP) lies under abductor pollicis brevis (AbPB).

C.   Adductor pollicis is a thenar muscle.

D.   All thenar muscles are supplied by the interosseous branch of the median nerve.

E.   OP inserts into the 1st metacarpal shaft.

True:	**A B E**
False:	**C D**

There are three thenar muscles: flexor pollicis brevis (FPB), AbPB, and OP, which all arise from
the flexor retinaculum. FPB and AbPB insert into the base of the proximal phalanx of the
thumb, and, respectively, flex and abduct the carpometacarpal (CMC) joint. OP lies deep to
these two muscles and inserts into the first metacarpal shaft. All are supplied by the recurrent
branch of the median nerve. Adductor pollicis attaches to the base of the proximal phalanx
of the thumb, and is not a thenar muscle as it is much more deeply placed. It has two bellies:
a transverse belly attaching to the middle metacarpal shaft; and an oblique belly attaching to
the capitate. Adductor pollicis is supplied by the ulnar nerve.

BLOOD SUPPLY

27. **The axillary artery.**

A. Is a continuation of the subclavian artery.

B. Gives a branch which supplies pectoralis major and minor.

C. Supplies the clavicle.

D. Is the only route through which blood enters the upper limb.

E. Terminates by dividing into the brachial artery and the profunda brachii artery.

True:	**A B C**
False:	**D E**

The axillary artery is a continuation of the subclavian artery as it passes over the first rib and it becomes the brachial artery as it passes the inferior border of teres major (this muscle defines the lower limit of the axilla). The axillary artery is crossed by pectoralis minor which divides the artery into three parts (1, 2 and 3 in *Figure 43*); conveniently, each part gives off 1, 2, and 3 branches, respectively (listed below).

1. Superior thoracic artery.

2. Acromiothoracic artery;
Lateral thoracic artery.

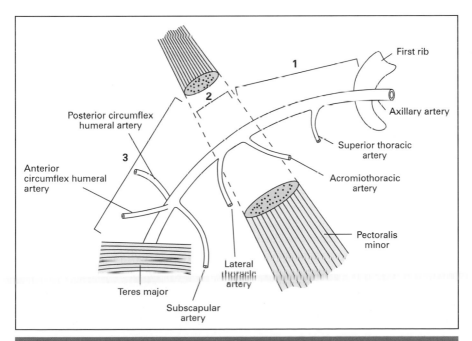

Fig. 43 The branches of the axillary artery. The axillary artery begins as a continuation of the subclavian artery as it passes over the first rib, and it continues as the brachial artery when it passes behind teres major. The overlying pectoralis minor conveniently divides the artery into its three parts (numbered 1, 2 and 3 in the diagram): note that the first part has 1 branch, the second part 2 branches, and the third part 3 branches.

3.   Subscapular artery;
     Anterior circumflex humeral artery;
     Posterior circumflex humeral artery.

The acromiothoracic trunk gives branches to the clavicle and the pectoral muscles. The subscapular artery gives off a circumflex scapular artery which forms an anastomosis around the scapula. This anastomosis includes branches from the subclavian artery (e.g., suprascapular artery and dorsal scapular artery), and is therefore an alternative route by which blood may reach the upper limb should the axillary artery become occluded.

28.   The brachial artery.

A.   Lies superficial to the deep fascia of the arm.

B.   Is accompanied by the brachial vein.

C.   Gives off four named branches before its termination.

D.   Usually crosses the median nerve.

E.   Gives off the common interrosseous artery.

True:	C
False:	A B D E

The brachial artery is a continuation of the axillary artery from the lower border of teres major, and it terminates by dividing into the ulnar and radial arteries at the level of the neck of the radius in the antecubital fossa. Despite running under the deep fascia of the arm, the brachial artery is a superficial structure that can be palpated just posterior to the belly of biceps. Although, in the majority (>80%) of cases, it is crossed by the median nerve from lateral to medial at the mid-point of the humerus, the artery may overlie the nerve. In addition to the nutrient artery to the humerus (given off half-way down the humerus), the brachial artery gives off three collateral branches: the profunda brachii artery; and superior and inferior ulnar collateral arteries. The profunda brachii artery is given off high up in the arm to the extensor compartment where it runs with the radial nerve in the spiral groove of the humerus before dividing into two terminal branches. These terminal branches, together with the two ulnar collateral branches, form an important anastomosis around the elbow joint with recurrent branches of the radial and ulnar arteries (their names deliberately omitted for the sake of simplicity). There is no brachial vein; the brachial artery is accompanied by paired venae commitantes.

29.   The radial and ulnar arteries in the forearm.

A.   The ulnar artery runs under FCU proximally.

B.   The radial artery runs under brachioradialis proximally.

C.   Distally the radial and ulnar arteries lie lateral to the tendons of flexor carpi radialis and FCU, respectively.

D. The common interosseous artery is usually a branch of the ulnar artery.

E. Both the radial artery and ulnar artery contribute to the dorsal and palmar carpal arches at the wrist.

All true.

In addition to the above, the following points are of note concerning the course of the radial and ulnar arteries and their branches in the forearm:

- The radial artery runs with the superficial radial nerve near the mid-point of the forearm; care must therefore be taken when ligating it in this region.

- The radial artery can be felt pulsating in the anatomical snuff-box (it gives off a branch here to the scaphoid).

- The common interosseous divides into anterior and posterior interosseous branches, which run on either side of the interosseous membrane between the radius and ulna.

30.   The arterial supply to the hand.

A. The radial artery gives rise to the superficial palmar arch.

B. The superficial palmar arch lies superficial to the palmar aponeurosis.

C. The deep palmar arch is more distal than the superficial palmar arch.

D. The thumb receives blood from the superficial palmar arch.

E. The palmar metacarpal arteries give rise to the palmar digital arteries.

All false.

The ulnar artery gives rise to the superficial palmar arch (most distal) which lies deep to the palmar aponeurosis. The deep carpal arch is derived from the radial artery after it pierces the first interosseous muscle. The superficial and deep arches are completed by communicating branches from the radial and ulnar arteries, respectively. The superficial arch gives rise to palmar digital arteries to the little, ring and middle fingers, and the ulnar half of the index finger, whereas the deep arch gives rise to the palmar digital branches to the thumb and remaining half of the index finger (respectively, princeps pollicis and radialis indicis arteries). The dorsal arch also gives rise to three palmar metacarpal arteries which, after supplying the small muscles of the hand and the metacarpal bones, anastomose with the palmar digital branches. Perforating branches from the palmar metacarpal arteries anastomose with the dorsal metacarpal arteries (these give rise to the dorsal digital arteries) which arise from the dorsal carpal arch.

31.   The venous drainage of the upper limb.

A. The cephalic vein drains into the brachial vein.

B. The basilic vein drains into the cephalic vein *via* the median cubital vein.

C. The basilic vein drains from the lateral part of the dorsal venous arch.

D. The cephalic vein drains from the superficial palmar venous arch.

E. The deep veins of the limb are paired and run with the arteries.

True:	E
False:	A B C D

The superficial veins of the upper limb are highly variable. There is a dorsal venous arch on the back of the hand (but no equivalent palmar arch) which drains laterally into the cephalic vein and medially into the basilic vein. The cephalic vein crosses the anatomical snuff-box and runs up the lateral side of the arm, communicating with the basilic vein by way of the median cubital vein at the antecubital fossa, before it pierces the deep fascia of the deltopectoral groove of the shoulder to join the axillary vein. The basilic vein pierces the deep fascia of the arm about half-way up the humerus to join with the venae commitantes (the paired deep veins) running with the brachial artery, to form the axillary vein (there is no brachial vein). In addition, there is often a small median vein on the anterior forearm that may drain into the cephalic, basilic, or median cubital veins. The lymphatic drainage of the upper limb follows the venous drainage to the axilla (*see* question on 'axilla'). There is one named node before the axilla: the supratrochlea node (sited with the basilic vein above the medial epicondyle of the humerus).

NEUROLOGY OF THE UPPER LIMB

32. **The nerve supply of muscles attaching the pectoral girdle to the trunk.**

Match each of the following muscles to the nerves given below. Each nerve may be used once, more than once, or not at all.

A. Levator scapulae

B. Serratus anterior

C. Pectoralis minor

D. Trapezius

E. Rhomboid major and minor

F. Subclavius

1. Long thoracic nerve

2. Dorsal scapular nerve

3. Axillary nerve

4. Thoracodorsal nerve

5. Suprascapular nerve

6. Accessory nerve (cranial XI)

7. None of the above nerves

Answers: A (2); B (1); C (7); D (6); E (2); F (7).

All the muscles attaching to the medial edge of the scapula (rhomboids and levator scapulae) are innervated by the dorsal scapular nerve. Serratus anterior attaches to the upper eight ribs and is supplied by the long thoracic nerve. The accessory nerve emerges from under sternocleidomastoid and crosses the posterior triangle of the neck to trapezius, and supplies both muscles (*see* Chapter 7, on the 'head and neck'). Both pectoralis major and minor are innervated by the medial and lateral pectoral nerves. Subclavius receives innervation from its own nerve (nerve to subclavius) which arises from the upper two roots (C5–C6) of the brachial plexus.

33. The components of the brachial plexus.

A. The brachial plexus has five roots beginning at C6.

B. The divisions are situated under the clavicle.

C. There are three posterior divisions.

D. The cords are situated in the axilla.

E. The median nerve receives fibres from the medial cord (MC) only.

True:	B C D
False:	A E

A plexus is the means by which segmental nerves are brought together to supply the muscles responsible for a given movement. The brachial plexus has important clinical significance because it can be damaged (trauma, cervical rib, tumour, surgery to root of the neck). At first glance the brachial plexus appears rather complex. However, it can be remembered using Reuben's rules of fives and threes.

- The plexus begins as five nerve roots (anterior primary rami).
- The first root is C5.
- The plexus ends as five main nerves to the upper limb (axillary, radial, musculocutaneous, median, radial, and ulnar).
- Between the roots and the main nerves there are: three trunks, three posterior divisions, three anterior divisions, and three cords.
- Including the five main terminal nerves, there is a total of 15 nerves arising from the plexus (conveniently remembered as 5 × 3 = 15!).

Figure 44A shows how fibres are distributed to the five main nerves of the upper limb: musculocutaneous nerve (C5, 6, 7); median nerve (C5, 6, 7, 8; T1); ulnar nerve (C8; T1); radial nerve (C5, 6, 7, 8; T1); axillary nerve (C5, 6). Note the sites of the roots, trunks, divisions and cords.

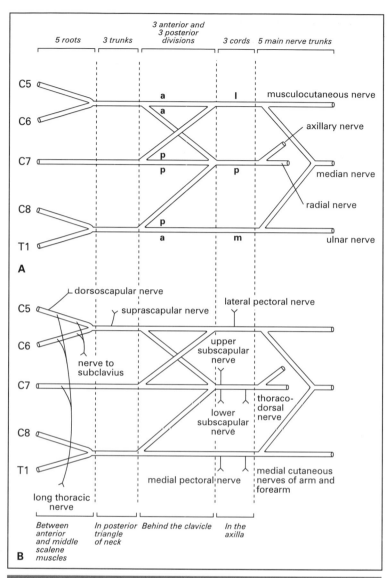

Fig. 44 A. Diagrammatic representation of the brachial plexus, excluding the small branches, showing the roots, trunks, divisions and cords. There are five main nerves to the upper limb; the plexus follows Reuben's rule of 5s and 3s. **a** = anterior; **p** = posterior; **l** = lateral; **m** = medial. **B.** The small branches of the brachial plexus.

34.   Small branches direct from the brachial plexus.

A.   The pectoral nerves arise from the medial and lateral trunks.

B.   The subscapular nerves arise from the posterior cord (PC).

C.   The long thoracic nerve arises in the neck.

D.   The dorsal scapular nerve arises from the lower cords.

E.   The thoracodorsal nerve is a branch of the PC.

True:	B C E
False:	A D

The 10 small nerves, that make up to 15 the total number of nerves arising directly from the plexus, are shown in *Figure 44B*. Some of the branches arise in the neck and some in the axilla. These branches and the muscles they innervate are listed below.

Branches arising in the neck (from roots and trunks)

- Dorsal scapular nerve (C5): levator scapular and rhomboids.
- Nerve to subclavius (C5, 6): subclavius.
- Long thoracic nerve of Bell (C5, 6, 7): serratus anterior.
- Suprascapular nerve (C5, 6): supraspinatus and infraspinatus.

Branches arising in the axilla (from cords)

- Upper subscapular nerve (C5, 6): subscapularis.
- Lower subscapular nerve (C5, 6): subscapularis and teres major.
- Thoracodorsal nerve (C5, 6, 7): latissimus dorsi.
- Lateral pectoral nerve (C5, 6): pectoralis major.
- Medial pectoral nerve (C8; T1): pectoralis major and minor.
- Medial cutaneous nerves of arm (T1) and forearm (C8).

35.   Brachial plexus injuries.

Match the following to either Erb's palsy or Klumpke's palsy.

A.   Upper brachial plexus lesion.

B.   Lower brachial plexus lesion.

C.   loss of shoulder abduction.

D.   Loss of the T1 segmental myotome.

E.   Paralysis of infraspinatus and teres minor.

F.   Loss of flexors of the wrist.

G.   Horner's syndrome.

H.   Loss of elbow flexion.

I.   Extension of the MCP joints and flexion of the interphalangeal (IP) joints.

J.   'Waiter's tip' position.

Erb's palsy:	A C E H J
Klumpke's palsy:	B D F G I

Erb's palsy

Erb's palsy is caused by injuries, particularly those sustained in motorcycle accidents, which jar the shoulder downwards. This stretches the upper roots of the brachial plexus (C5, 6) and thereby produces paralysis of the suprascapular nerve, the musculocutaneous nerve and axillary nerve:

- Loss of shoulder abduction: deltoid and supraspinatus.
- Loss of external rotation of the shoulder: infraspinatus and teres major.
- Loss of elbow flexion: biceps, brachialis and brachioradialis.
- Loss of supination of forearm: biceps (most powerful supinator).

The upper limb is held with the shoulder adducted and internally rotated, the elbow extended, and forearm pronated. This is known as the 'Waiter's tip' position.

Klumpke's palsy

Klumpke's palsy is caused by injuries where the shoulder is abducted, e.g., in a breech birth. The lower fibres of the brachial plexus are damaged, causing a T1 segmental paralysis. T1 is the segmental myotome to all the small muscles of the hand through the median and ulnar nerves. This leads to unopposed action of the long flexors and extensors. The IP joints are therefore held flexed and the MCP joints extended.

36.	The musculocutaneous nerve.

A. Arises from the lateral cord (LC) of the brachial plexus.

B. Pierces pectoralis minor.

C. Runs lateral to coracobrachialis.

D. Runs between biceps and brachialis.

E. Innervates skin of the medial forearm.

True:	A
False:	B C D E

The musculocutaneous nerve arises from the LC of the brachial plexus, and pierces coracobrachialis before running beneath biceps and brachialis. It supplies all three of these muscles and is therefore responsible for flexion of the elbow. It terminates by supplying skin on the lateral side of the forearm.

37.	The axillary nerve.

A. Arises from the PC of the brachial plexus.

B. Passes through the QS.

C. Is closely related to the surgical neck of the humerus.

D. Supplies teres major.

E. Supplies skin over the 'badge' area overlying deltoid.

True:	A B C E
False:	D

The axillary nerve supplies deltoid and teres minor. Its close relation to the surgical neck means that it is prone to injury in fractures at this site and also when the humeral head dislocates. The integrity of the axillary nerve can be tested in the injured subject by examining sensation over the so-called 'badge' area of skin, as the axillary nerve gives rise to the upper lateral cutaneous nerve of the arm.

38.   The radial nerve.

A.   Arises from the PC of the brachial plexus.

B.   Damage to the nerve in the spiral groove causes loss of elbow extension and wrist drop.

C.   Damage to the posterior interosseus branch causes wrist drop alone.

D.   Damage to the superficial radial nerve causes sensory loss over the greater part of the dorsum of the hand.

E.   The radial nerve only supplies extensor muscles.

True:	A
False:	B C D E

The radial nerve arises from the PC of the brachial plexus, and passes posterior to the axillary artery between the long and medial heads of triceps, to lie in the spiral groove between medial and lateral heads of triceps. Here, it is accompanied by the profunda brachii artery before it pierces the lateral intermuscular septum at the lower third of the humerus to run between brachialis and brachioradialis. At the level of the lateral epicondyle of the humerus, it gives rise to the posterior interosseus nerve and the superficial radial nerve. The posterior interosseus is the larger of these two branches and should really be considered to be a continuation of the muscular component of the radial nerve in the forearm. The radial nerve supplies all the extensors of the arm and forearm. However, it also supplies brachioradialis, which is a flexor of the elbow joint when the forearm is pronated. Damage to the nerve in the spiral groove causes wrist drop but not loss of elbow extension, as fibres to triceps remain intact proximal to this site. Only damage in the axilla will cause loss of elbow extension and wrist drop. Damage to the posterior interosseus branch does not cause wrist drop because extensor carpi radialis longus receives its innervation from the main radial nerve. Although the superficial radial nerve does supply sensation to the skin over the dorsum of the hand, damage results only in loss of sensation in the first dorsal web space due to overlap in innervation from the median and ulnar nerves.

39.   The median nerve.

A.   Passes lateral to the brachial artery throughout the arm.

B.   Passes between the heads of pronator teres.

C.   Damage at the elbow results in loss of pronation of the forearm.

D.   'Monkey-hand' is a good description of the position of the hand in median nerve damage.

E.   Carpal tunnel syndrome results in sensation loss in the lateral three and a half fingers and over the thenar eminence.

True:	B C D
False:	A E

The median nerve arises from the lateral and MC of the brachial plexus. It passes lateral to the brachial artery before passing underneath it to run medially (it may pass over the artery in some individuals). The nerve enters the forearm between the heads of pronator teres, and at this point gives off its anterior interosseus branch. The median nerve continues throughout the forearm adherent to the undersurface of FDS and passes through the carpal tunnel. The median nerve supplies no muscles in the upper arm, but in the forearm it supplies all muscles in the flexor aspect of the forearm apart from FCU and the ulnar half of flexor digitorum profundus. In the hand, it supplies the thenar muscles and the radial two lumbricals. As it supplies pronator teres and pronator quadratus, damage to the nerve above the elbow, e.g., in supracondylar fractures, results in loss of pronation of the forearm. Paralysis of the thenar muscles causes the palm to lie flatter than normal giving the appearance of a 'monkey-hand'. The median nerve supplies sensation to the lateral three and a half digits and to the thenar eminence. However, sensation over the thenar eminence is spared in carpal tunnel syndrome, because the palmar cutaneous branch does not pass through the carpal tunnel.

40.   The ulnar nerve.

A.   Passes deep to triceps.

B.   Passes behind the medial epicondyle.

C.   Lies beneath FCU in the proximal forearm.

D.   Injury at the wrist causes loss of thumb adduction.

E.   Injury at the wrist causes loss of any extension of the little- and ring-finger IP joints.

True:	A B C D
False:	E

The ulnar nerve supplies FCU, the ulnar half of flexor digitorum profundus, and all the intrinsic muscles of the hand except those of the thenar eminence and the radial two lumbricals. Injury to the nerve at the wrist will therefore cause a weakness in the intrinsic muscles but not flexor digitorum profundus. This results in the ulnar 'claw' where the little- and ring-finger IP joints are flexed and the metacarpophalangeal joints of the same are more extended. Extension of the fingers is not completely lost, however, because of the action of the long extensors of the fingers. The ulnar claw can therefore be understood as lack of compensation for flexor digitorum profundus on the little- and ring-fingers due to paralysis of the intrinsic muscles. The radial two lumbricals are supplied by the median nerve and so the index and middle fingers are spared.

5. Lower Limb

TOPIC CHECK LIST

IMPORTANT REGIONS OF THE LOWER LIMB

1. The femoral triangle.

A. Sartorius forms its medial wall, and adductor brevis its lateral wall.

B. Fascia lata forms its roof.

C. The great saphenous vein enters the triangle at its most inferior angle.

D. The femoral triangle contains the lateral cutaneous nerve of the thigh.

E. The femoral triangle contains the deep inguinal lymph nodes.

True:	B D E
False:	**A C**

The femoral triangle (*Figure 45*) is bounded by the inguinal ligament superiorly, sartorius laterally, and adductor longus medially. Its floor is formed by iliopsoas and pectineus. It is roofed over by the fascia lata, which is the deep fascia of the lower limb. Above the fascia lata is the superficial fascia, which contains superficial inguinal lymph nodes and the great saphenous vein. The great saphenous vein pierces the fascia lata at its saphenous opening to join the femoral vein.

In addition

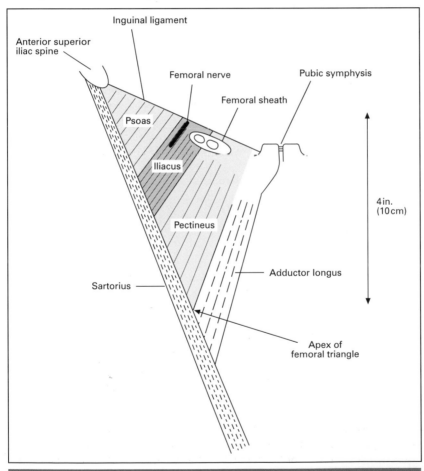

Fig. 45 Diagrammatic representation of the borders (inguinal ligament, sartorius, and adductor longus) and the floor of the femoral triangle. The femoral sheath (enclosing the femoral artery and femoral vein) and the femoral nerve are shown entering the femoral triangle underneath the inguinal ligament. The triangle is 4 in. (10 cm) long from the inguinal ligament to its apex.

to the femoral vein, the triangle contains the femoral nerve and artery: remember VAN (vein/artery/nerve) from medial to lateral. All three structures enter the femoral triangle under the inguinal ligament, and the pulse of the femoral artery can be felt at the mid-inguinal point. The lateral cutaneous nerve of the thigh also passes under the inguinal ligament to lie in the lateral corner of the triangle. The femoral triangle also contains the deep inguinal nodes.

2.   The saphenous opening in the anterior thigh.

A.   Is an opening in the fascia lata.

B.   Is situated 4 cm below and lateral to the pubic symphysis.

C.   Transmits the great saphenous vein.

D.   Transmits the femoral artery.

E.   The falciform margin lies superiorly.

True:	A C
False:	B D E

The saphenous opening is a gap in the fascia lata, covered by loose connective tissue called the cribriform fascia. It is situated 1½ in. (4 cm) below and lateral to the pubic tubercle. The lower lateral border of the opening is known as the falciform margin. In addition to the great saphenous vein, the following branches and tributaries of the femoral vessels pass through the saphenous opening (lateral to medial): superficial circumflex iliac artery and vein; superficial epigastric artery and vein; superficial external pudendal vessels.

3.   The femoral canal.

A.   It serves no known function, but is important clinically as a site of herniation of the small bowel.

B.   It is surrounded by the femoral sheath on all sides.

C.   It contains the femoral nerve.

D.   It contains a lymph node called Cloquet's node.

E.   The femoral vein lies medially.

True:	D
False:	A B C E

The femoral sheath is a fascial tube derived from extra-peritoneal intraabdominal fascia. It extends under the inguinal ligament to surround the femoral vessels. The femoral canal is a small space (approximately 1¼ in. or 0.5 cm wide) between the medial part of the sheath and the femoral vein (*see Figure 46*). It contains a fat plug and Cloquet's lymph node. The canal serves as a pathway for lower limb lymphatics and allows for expansion of the femoral vessels. Femoral hernias can be differentiated from inguinal hernias by locating the neck of femoral hernia below and lateral to the inguinal canal.

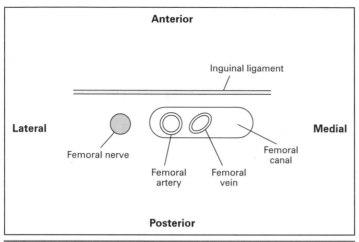

Anterior

Inguinal ligament

Lateral

Femoral nerve

Femoral artery

Femoral vein

Femoral canal

Medial

Posterior

Fig. 46 Cross-section of the right femoral nerve, artery and vein, as seen from below as they pass under the inguinal ligament. It can be seen that the femoral sheath surrounds the femoral vessels, leaving a space, known as the femoral canal, medial to the vein. The femoral nerve lies laterally, outside the femoral sheath.

4. The adductor canal of Hunter.

A. Contains the saphenous nerve.

B. Contains the sciatic nerve.

C. Contains the femoral nerve.

D. Is roofed by sartorius.

E. Is approximately 25 cm long.

True:	A D
False:	B C E

The inferior outlet of the femoral triangle becomes roofed over by sartorius (the most superficial muscle of the anterior thigh) to form an intermuscular tunnel approximately 6 in. (15 cm) long, known as the adductor canal of Hunter (it is named after John Hunter who described the exposure and ligation of the femoral artery for treatment of popliteal aneurysm). The canal contains the femoral vessels and a branch of the femoral nerve, the saphenous nerve. The canal terminates at the adductor hiatus (an opening in the adductor magnus muscle) where the femoral vessels pass posteriorly into the popliteal fossa behind the knee joint. Including its passage through the femoral triangle, therefore, the femoral artery runs a total course of 10 in. (25 cm) in the anterior thigh.

5. The popliteal fossa.

A. It is bounded laterally by biceps femoris and gastrocnemius.

B. Its roof is pierced by the short saphenous vein.

C. The popliteal artery is the deepest structure in the fossa.

D. The common peroneal (fibular) nerve runs along its medial border.

E. The popliteal vein runs superficial to the tibial nerve (TN).

True:	A B C
False:	D E

The popliteal fossa (*Figure 47*) is a diamond-shaped area behind the knee, bounded by the hamstrings above (biceps femoris laterally) and the two heads of gastrocnemius below. Like the femoral triangle, the popliteal fossa is roofed over by a deep fascia. Unlike the femoral triangle, however, the deep fascia of the popliteal fossa is pierced by the short saphenous vein, as opposed to the great saphenous vein. In addition to lymph nodes and fat, the fossa contains (from superficial to deep): the branches of the sciatic nerve; the popliteal vein (receiving the short saphenous vein); and the popliteal artery (being deep, the popliteal pulse is notoriously difficult to palpate). The sciatic nerve divides into the tibial and common peroneal (fibular) nerves. The common peroneal nerve lies laterally in the fossa along the medial border of the biceps femoris.

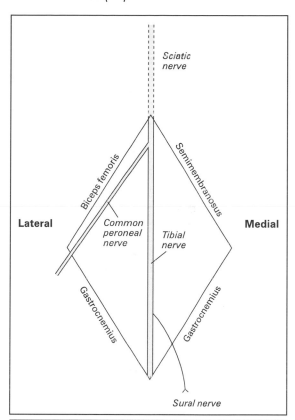

Fig. 47 Muscular boundaries of the popliteal fossa, and the divisions of the sciatic nerve into the tibial nerve (TN) and the common parietal nerve. The TN gives rise to the sacral nerve.

MUSCULAR COMPARTMENTS AND INNERVATION OF THE LOWER LIMB

6.   The muscular compartments of the thigh.

A. There are four muscular compartments formed by fibrous septae passing from the femur to the fascia lata.

B. The obturator nerve supplies the posterior compartment.

C. The posterior compartment is supplied by the sciatic nerve.

D. Adductor magnus lies in the posterior compartment.

E. Tensor fasciae latae is part of the lateral (gluteal) compartment.

True:	C
False:	A B D E

There are three compartments to the thigh, formed by the three septae passing from the femur to the fascia lata: anterior, posterior and medial compartments. There is no lateral compartment as such. The three compartments and their nerve supply, are shown diagrammatically in Figure 48.

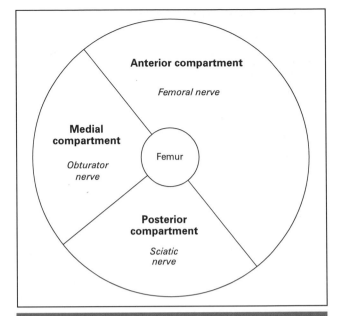

Fig. 48 Diagram showing the three compartments of the thigh and their nerve supply.

Medial thigh

(Obturator nerve L2–L4)

- Pectineus*
- Adductor longus
- Adductor magnus**
- Adductor brevis
- Gracilis
- Obturator externus

Anterior thigh

(Femoral nerve L2–L4)

- Psoas
- Iliacus
- Tensor fasciae latae***
- Sartorius
- Quadriceps femoris (Rectus and Vastii)

Posterior thigh

(Sciatic nerve L4, 5; S1–S3)

- Semimembranosus
- Semitendinosus
- Biceps femoris

Special cases:

   * Pectineus   – dual supply from the obturator and femoral nerves.

  ** Adductor magnus   – dual supply from the obturator and sciatic nerves.

*** Tensor fasciae latae – superior gluteal nerve.

---

7. The muscles of the anterior thigh.

A. Rectus femoris extends the hip joint.

B. Sartorius flexes the hip and knee joint.

C. Vastus intermedialis is supplied by the obturator nerve.

D. The lowest fibres of vastus medialis insert into the patella lower than the lateral fibres.

E. The anterior thigh muscles are supplied by the brachial artery.

F. Psoas inserts into the greater trochanter.

G. Tensor fasciae latae is supplied by the inferior gluteal nerve.

H. The femoral nerve supplies iliacus.

I. Iliacus and psoas pass from the floor of the femoral triangle.

J. Iliacus extends the hip joint.

True:	**B D H I**
False:	**A C E F G J**

The muscles of the anterior thigh include psoas, iliacus, tensor fasciae latae, sartorius and quadriceps femoris (rectus femoris, vastus medialis, vastus lateralis and vastus intermedius). Rectus femoris arises from the anterior inferior iliac spine, the vastus medialis and lateralis muscles arise from the linea aspera of the femur, and vastus intermedius arises from the anterior and lateral surfaces of the shaft of the femur. The quadriceps muscles insert into the patella, which attaches to the tibial tuberosity *via* the patellar tendon, and extend the knee joint. Rectus femoris is also a weak flexor of the hip. Sartorius arises from the ASIS and inserts into the proximal part of the medial tibia. Sartorius means 'tailor's muscle' and refers to its action in crossing the legs (flexing the hip and knee, abducting and laterally rotating the hip) because the crossed leg position was associated with tailors. Quadriceps femoris and sartorius are supplied by the femoral nerve (L2, L3, L4). Blood supply to the thigh is from profunda femoris, a branch of the femoral artery.

Psoas arises from the sides of T12–L5 vertebrae, discs and transverse processes. Iliacus arises from the iliac crest and fossa. Iliacus and psoas insert into the lesser trochanter and flex the hip joint. Tensor fasciae latae originates from the anterior part of the iliac crest, ASIS and inserts into the iliotibial tract, which attaches to the lateral condyle of the tibia. It keeps the knee extended when standing, and is supplied by the superior gluteal nerve.

8. The muscles of the posterior thigh.

A. The tendon of biceps femoris inserts into the head of the fibula.

B. Semitendinosus is supplied by the tibial division of the sciatic nerve.

C. The hamstring muscles extend the hip.

D. The short head of biceps arises from the ischial tuberosity.

E. The semimembranosus inserts into the proximal end of the lateral tibia.

True:	**A B C**
False:	**D E**

The muscles of the posterior thigh include semitendinosus, semimembranosus and biceps femoris. Semitendinosus, semimembranosus and the long head of biceps femoris arise from the ischial tuberosity and are supplied by the tibial division of the sciatic nerve (L4–S3). The short head of biceps femoris arises from the linea aspera and lateral supracondylar line of the femur, and is supplied by the common fibular division of the sciatic nerve. Semitendinosus and semimembranosus insert into the proximal medial tibia. The tendon of biceps femoris inserts into the head of the fibula; it is split by the lateral collateral ligament of the knee. The hamstring muscles extend the hip and flex the knee. With the leg flexed, biceps femoris may rotate the leg laterally, while semitendinosus and semimembranosus can rotate the leg medially on the thigh.

9. The muscles of the medial thigh.

A. Gracilis inserts into the medial condyle of the femur.

B. The adductor hiatus is an opening in the lower end of the adductor magnus muscle.

C. Adductor brevis, longus and magnus all insert into the linea aspera.

D. Pectineus inserts into the lesser trochanter.

E. The muscles of the medial thigh are supplied by the lesser gluteal nerve.

True:	B C
False:	A D E

The muscles of the medial (adductor) compartment fan out from their origins on the front of the pubic and ischial bones to insert along the length of the femur. Pectineus has the highest attachment to the femur on the pectineal line, just below the lesser trochanter. Adductor brevis, longus and magnus all insert into the linea aspera, although only magnus attaches its full length and extends along the medial supracondylar line and to the adductor tubercle. There is a gap in magnus, just above the adductor tubercle, known as the adductor hiatus, which allows for passage of the femoral vessels to the popliteal fossa posteriorly. Gracilis, the most medial of the adductor muscles, has no attachment to the femur, but crosses the knee to insert into the medial surface of the tibia. All the muscles are innervated by the obturator nerve, with contributions from the femoral nerve to pectineus, and from the sciatic nerve to adductor magnus.

10. The gluteal region.

A. Gluteus maximus is supplied by the superior gluteal nerve.

B. Gluteus maximus inserts into the greater trochanter of the femur.

C. The sciatic nerve frequently passes into the gluteal region through the greater sciatic foramen above the piriformis muscle.

D. The deep muscles of this region (piriformis, gemilli, obturator internus, and quadratus femoris) all laterally rotate the hip by pulling on their insertion into the greater trochanter of the femur.

E. The posterior cutaneous nerve of the thigh lies medial to the sciatic nerve.

True:	E
False:	A B C D

The muscles of the gluteal region consist of the glutei (maximus, medius and minimis) and the deep lateral rotators of the hip (piriformis, gemelli, obturator internus, and quadratus femoris). All the glutei extend and abduct the hip. Gluteus medius and minimis attach, respectively, to the lateral and anterior surfaces of the greater trochanter, and are both

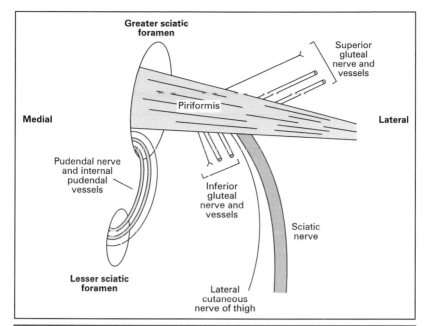

Fig. 49 Diagrammatic representation of the NV structures of the right gluteal region, summarising how these structures are related to the piriformis muscle which passes out from the pelvis through the greater sciatic foramen.

supplied by the superior gluteal nerve (L5; S1). It is damage to this nerve, which also supplies tensor fasciae latae in the anterior compartment, that gives rise to a Trendelenburg gait (inability to support the pelvis when standing on one leg, causing the pelvis to dip on the opposite side). The upper ¼ fibres of gluteus maximus insert into the gluteal tuberosity of the femur and the lower ¾ fibres insert into the iliotibial tract. Gluteus maximus is supplied by the inferior gluteal nerve (L5; S1). Almost all the deep lateral rotators of the hip insert into the medial surface of the greater trochanter, except for quadratus femoris which inserts into the quadrate tubercle below. The nerve supply to the lateral rotators is summarised below.

Nerve supply to lateral rotators of hip

- Piriformis: ventral rami of S1, 2.

- Obturator internus: nerve to obturator internus (L5; S1).

- Superior gemellus: nerve to obturator internus (L5; S1).

- Inferior gemellus: nerve to quadratus femoris (L5; S1).

- Quadratus femoris: nerve to quadratus femoris (L5; S1).

Figure 49 shows the relationship of various structures in the gluteal region. Note that the piriformis muscle is an important landmark for identifying structures passing out of the greater sciatic foramen, the superior gluteal vessels and nerves passing above piriformis and the inferior passing below. Although, in most cases, the sciatic nerve passes below the piriformis, with the posterior cutaneous nerve to the thigh, it may also pass through it (10% of cases) or above it (<1% of cases).

---

11.   The muscular compartments of the lower leg.

A.   Anterior and a posterior fascial septa join the fibula to the deep fascia of the leg and divide the lower leg into three compartments.

B.   The interosseus membrane joins the tibia and fibula between the anterior and lateral compartments.

C.   Soleus is deep to the deep transverse fascia in the posterior compartment.

D.   Extensor digitorum longus is part of the lateral compartment.

E.   FDL is part of the lateral compartment.

True:	A
False:	B C D E

There are three muscular compartments in the lower leg, anterior, posterior and lateral (peroneal/fibular). They are divided by the interosseus membrane (between anterior and posterior compartments) and the anterior and posterior fascial septa attached to the fibula. Furthermore, the posterior compartment is divided into superficial and deep parts by the deep transverse fascia. A diagrammatic representation of the compartments, the contained muscles, and their nerve supply, is shown in *Figure 50*.

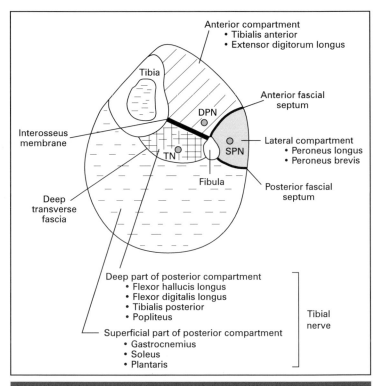

Fig. 50 Diagrammatic summary of the muscles and innervation of the fascial compartments of the lower leg. DPN = deep peroneal nerve; SPN = superficial peroneal nerve; TN = tibial nerve.

Posterior compartment

(TN, L4–S3)

Deep muscles

- Tibialis posterior
- FDL
- Flexor hallucis longus
- Popliteus

Superficial muscles

- Gastrocnemius
- Plantaris
- Soleus

Anterior compartment

(Deep peroneal nerve [DPN], L4–S2)

- Tibialis anterior
- Extensor digitorum longus
- Extensor hallucis longus

Lateral compartment

(Superficial peroneal nerve [SPN], L5–S2)

- Peroneus longus
- Peroneus brevis

---

12.   The muscles of the lateral (peroneal) compartment of the lower leg.

A.   Behind the lateral malleolus, the tendon of peroneus brevis is below that of peroneus longus.

B.   Peroneus longus, but not brevis, attaches to the tibia.

C.   Peroneus longus inserts into the medial cuneiform and the 1st metatarsal.

D.   Peroneus brevis inserts into the 5th metatarsal.

E.   The tendons of the peroneal muscles pass under the extensor retinaculum.

True:	C D
False:	A B E

There are two muscles in the lateral, or peroneal (fibular) compartment: peroneus brevis and longus. Both arise from the lateral surface of the fibula (brevis from the lower 2/3 and longus from the upper 1/3) and this is why they carry the name peroneus, which means 'of the fibula'. Both tendons pass under the peroneal retinaculum behind the lower end of the fibula (brevis superior to longus). While brevis inserts directly into the 5th metatarsal on the lateral side of the foot, longus passes medially to the 1st metatarsal and the medial cuneiform on the medial side of the foot. Both muscles are supplied by the SPN, both evert the foot, and longus also plantarflexes the foot. The medial cuneiform has important attachments from lower leg muscles. It also provides attachments for both tibialis anterior and tibialis posterior.

---

13.   The muscles of the anterior compartment of the lower leg.

A.   All the muscles of the anterior compartment of the leg dorsiflex the foot.

B.   Tibialis anterior inserts into the 1st metatarsal.

C.   Tibialis anterior inverts the foot.

D. Peroneus tertius attaches to the base of the 5th metatarsal.

E. Extensor digitorum longus arises from the front of the fibula.

All true.

There are three muscles in the anterior compartment of the lower leg; all send tendons under the extensor retinaculum and all dorsiflex the foot. In addition, tibialis anterior, which arises from the shaft of the tibia and inserts into the 1st metatarsal and medial cuneiform, will invert the foot. The two long extensors of the toes arise from the front of the fibula. Extensor hallucis longus sends its tendon to the distal phalanx of the great toe and extensor digitorum longus sends out four tendons to the distal phalanges of the other four toes. Peroneus tertius is a small accessory muscle arising from extensor digitorum longus and inserts into the base of the 5th metatarsal. All the muscles of the anterior compartment are innervated by the DPN.

14. The muscles of the posterior compartment of the lower leg.

A. Gastrocnemius has a single head from the lateral condyle of the femur.

B. Soleus lies superficial to plantaris.

C. Soleus inserts into the talus.

D. Behind the medial malleolus the tendon of flexor hallucis longus lies most anterior.

E. The tendons of FDL insert into the middle phalanges.

All false.

The three superficial muscles of the posterior compartment (gastrocnemius, plantaris, and soleus) are equivalent to the triceps surae muscle found in many other mammals. They all have a common insertion through the Achille's tendon into the calcaneus. Gastrocnemius has two heads arising from each of the femoral condyles, while soleus arises from the soleal line of the tibia: both these muscles are powerful plantar flexors of the foot, whereas the plantaris muscle is rudimentary. The deep muscles of the posterior compartment include: popliteus; tibialis posterior; and the long flexors of the toes. Popliteus passes inside the capsule of the knee joint and has a role in 'unlocking' the knee (*see* Question 29 of this chapter on movements of the knee joint). Tibialis posterior is a plantar flexor of the foot. The long flexors of the toes (flexor hallucis and digitorum longus) mirror the long flexors of the fingers and insert into the distal phalanges. The order of structures running under the flexor retinaculum behind the medial malleolus can be remembered by the mnemonic 'Timothy Doth Vex All Nervous Housewives' as (from front to back): **T**ibialis posterior, flexor **D**igitorum longus, tibial **V**ein, **A**rtery, **N**erve, and flexor **H**allucis longus.

15. The cutaneous innervation of the lower limb.

A. The lateral, intermediate and cutaneous nerves are all branches of the femoral nerve.

B. Skin below the inguinal ligament medial to sartorius is supplied by branches of the femoral nerve.

C. The saphenous nerve supplies skin on the medial side of the lower leg.

D. The posterior cutaneous nerve of the thigh runs under the fascia lata.

E.   The lateral sides of the feet are innervated by S1.

F.   The sural nerve is a branch of the common peroneal nerve.

G.   The SPN supplies all the skin on the dorsal surface of the foot.

True:	A C D E
False:	B F G

On the anterior thigh, skin lateral to the sartorius muscle is supplied by three cutaneous branches of the femoral nerve (lateral, intermediate and medial cutaneous nerves of the thigh). The saphenous nerve is also a cutaneous branch of the femoral nerve, but it passes through the adductor canal of Hunter to supply skin more distal to the thigh on the medial side of the lower leg, and onto the foot as far as the head of the first metatarsal. All these cutaneous branches of the femoral nerve form a patellar plexus in front of the knee. On the anterior thigh, medial to the line of sartorius, and below the inguinal ligament, skin is not supplied by the femoral nerve but by the ilioinguinal nerve and the femoral branch of the genito-femoral nerve. The medial aspect of the thigh receives innervation from the obturator nerve. The posterior cutaneous nerve of the thigh is a branch of the sacral plexus that enters the thigh through the greater sciatic foramen below piriformis and medial to the sciatic nerve; it then runs under the fascia lata, giving numerous branches to the overlying skin before becoming superficial in the popliteal fossa, where it terminates. The sural nerve is a branch of the TN, although it receives a communicating branch from the common peroneal nerve. The sural nerve provides innervation to the posterior and lateral sides of the lower leg and supplies the lateral side of the foot, including the lateral aspect of the little toe. The sole of the foot is innervated by branches of the TN, while the dorsum of the foot is innervated by the SPN, except for the first dorsal web space which is innervated by the DPN.

16.   Nerve injuries in the lower limb.

Match the following clinical features to injury of the appropriate nerves listed below.

A.   Paralysis of the hamstrings and all muscles below the knee, and associated loss of sensation below the knee, except on the medial side down as far as the big toe.

B.   Plantar-flexion and inversion of the foot.

C.   Loss of knee extension and loss of sensation on the medial side of the lower part of the leg as far as the big toe.

D.   Loss of sensation in the first dorsal web space of the foot.

E.   Loss of sensation on the sole of the foot.

1.   TN

2.   DPN

3.   Femoral nerve

4.   Sciatic nerve

5.   Common peroneal nerve

Answers: A (4); B (5); C (3); D (2); E (1).

Note that the saphenous nerve, which is a branch of the femoral nerve, supplies sensation on the medial side of the lower leg and foot down as far as the big toe.

BLOOD SUPPLY OF THE LOWER LIMB

17. The femoral artery and its branches.

A. The femoral artery enters the thigh under the inguinal ligament at its mid-point.

B. The medial and lateral circumflex femoral arteries are direct branches of the femoral artery.

C. The femoral artery always lies lateral to the femoral vein.

D. The femoral artery is separated from the hip joint by psoas.

E. The femoral artery gives off a single descending branch to the knee joint.

True:	D E
False:	A B C

The femoral artery is approximately 10 in. (25 cm) long and enters the thigh under the inguinal ligament at the mid-inguinal point (half-way between the pubic symphysis and the ASIS, not the mid-point of the inguinal ligament). The artery runs through the femoral triangle and adductor canal before passing through the adductor hiatus to become the popliteal artery. The psoas muscle separates the femoral artery from the hip joint posteriorly. The femoral vein lies medial to the artery in the femoral sheath, but then passes behind to become lateral at the level of the adductor tubercle. As it passes under the inguinal ligament, the femoral artery almost immediately gives off several small branches to: the abdominal wall (superficial epigastric); the external genitalia (external pudendal arteries); and the anterior thigh (superficial circumflex iliac artery). The main branch of the femoral artery is, however, the profunda femoris (deep femoral artery), which gives rise to the lateral and medial circumflex femoral arteries. The most distal branch of the femoral artery is the descending genicular artery to the knee joint.

18. The profunda femoris artery and its branches.

A. The profunda femoris lies deep to adductor magnus.

B. There is an anastomosis with the inferior gluteal artery.

C. There are five perforating branches.

D. The perforating branches all pass through adductor magnus.

E. The lateral circumflex femoral artery passes posterior to the femur.

True:	B D
False:	A C E

The profunda femoris is the largest branch of the femoral artery and arises from its lateral side about 4 cm below the inguinal ligament. It gives off the medial and lateral circumflex femoral arteries at its origin, and these pass posterior and anterior to the femur, respectively. The profunda dives deep to adductor longus to lie in the medial compartment of the thigh. Here, it gives off three perforating branches before terminating as the fourth perforator. All the perforators pass through the adductor magnus muscle to supply the posterior compartment of the thigh. There is a longitudinal anastomosis between all the posterior perforators which also communicates with the inferior gluteal artery (this provides an alternative route for blood to the lower limb if the femoral artery is occluded).

19. The arterial supply of the lower leg and foot.

A. The peroneal artery is a branch of the anterior tibial artery.

B. The peroneal artery runs in the posterior compartment of the lower leg.

C. The pulse of the posterior tibial artery can be felt in front of the medial malleolus.

D. The pulse of dorsalis pedis can be felt between the 4th and 5th metatarsals.

E. The medial and lateral plantar arteries are branches of the posterior tibial artery.

True:	B E
False:	A C D

The popliteal artery divides into anterior and posterior tibial arteries as it passes under the fibrous arch of soleus, about a hand's breadth below the knee. The anterior tibial artery passes forward over the interosseus membrane, upon which it then descends (supplies the anterior compartment of the lower leg) to cross the ankle joint mid-way between the malleoli. It passes under the extensor retinacula and becomes the dorsalis pedis artery. The dorsalis pedis pulse can be felt between the metatarsals of the great and 2nd toes before it terminates by dividing into dorsal digital branches. The peroneal arises from the posterior tibial artery approximately 1 in. (2.5 cm) below its origin under soleus. It then runs in the posterior compartment between the tibialis posterior muscle and the flexor hallucis longus muscle and supplies the lateral (peroneal) compartment through lateral branches. The peroneal artery divides into its small terminal branches at the level of the inferior tibiofibular joint. The posterior tibial artery supplies the muscles of the posterior compartment as it passes through it. It can be palpated posterior to the medial malleolus. It passes under the flexor retinaculum before bifurcating into the medial and lateral plantar arteries.

20. The venous drainage of the lower limb.

A. The small saphenous vein drains directly into the femoral vein.

B. The great saphenous vein accompanies the saphenous artery.

C. The small saphenous vein begins at the medial end of the dorsal venous arch of the foot.

D. There is no communication between the small and great saphenous veins above the ankle.

E. The great saphenous vein passes in front of the medial malleolus.

True:	E
False:	A B C D

As in the upper limb, there are paired venae commitantes that accompany the small arteries of the lower limb. The superficial veins of the lower limb consist of the great and small saphenous veins. The small saphenous vein drains from the lateral end of the dorsal venous arch of the foot and drains into the popliteal vein in the popliteal fossa. The great saphenous vein drains from the medial end of the dorsal venous arch of the foot and passes anterior to the medial malleolus, then up the lower leg to pass about a hand's breadth behind the patella before traversing the medial thigh to the saphenous opening in the fascia lata, where it dives deep to join the femoral vein. There are many perforating veins between the deep and superficial veins of the lower limb. These perforators contain valves to prevent flow from deep to superficial veins and it is incompetence of these valves that causes varicose veins. The constant anterior relation of the great saphenous vein to the medial malleolus is essential to remember, as it is a useful site to perform a cut-down for an emergency blood transfusion.

JOINTS OF THE LOWER LIMB

21. The normal anatomy of the hip joint.

A.   The hip is a hinge joint.

B.   The iliofemoral ligament prevents overextension of the hip.

C.   The capsule of the hip joint completely covers the neck of the femur.

D.   Quadratus femoris is a lateral rotator of the hip.

E.   Psoas major lies medial to the hip joint.

True:	B D
False:	A C E

The hip joint is a synovial ball-and-socket joint between the hemispherical head of the femur and the cup-shaped acetabulum of the innominate (hip) bone. The acetabulum has a central depression known as the acetabular fossa, surrounded by a horseshoe-shaped articular surface, which is deficient inferiorly at the acetabular notch. The cavity of the acetabulum is deepened by the acetabular labrum, and where this crosses the acetabular notch it is known as the transverse acetabular ligament. The capsule of the hip joint attaches to the acetabular labrum and passes to the intertrochanteric line of the femur anteriorly. Posteriorly, it attaches to the neck of the femur above the intertrochanteric crest. The capsule is reinforced by three ligaments: the Y-shaped iliofemoral ligament; the triangular shaped pubofemoral ligament; and the spiral-shaped ischiofemoral ligament. Within the hip joint, stretching between the transverse ligament and a small pit on the head of the femur (the fovea), is the ligament of the head of the femur. This being a synovial joint, the articular surfaces are covered with hyaline cartilage and a synovial membrane lines the inside of the joint. This synovial lining covers a fat pad in the acetabular fossa, surrounds the ligament of the head of the femur, and may protrude through the anterior capsule between the pubofemoral and iliofemoral ligaments to form the psoas bursa (which lies beneath the tendon of psoas major). The blood supply to the hip joint is from the obturator artery (which gives a branch to the head of the femur through the ligament of the head of the femur), the medial and lateral circumflex femoral arteries (both arise from the profunda femoris artery), and the nutrient artery of the femur. Sensory nerve supply to the hip is from the femoral, obturator, and sciatic nerves. The femoral nerve is separated from the hip joint anteriorly by the iliopsoas and rectus femoris muscles. The sciatic nerve is separated from the hip joint posteriorly by the lateral rotators of the hip: quadratus femoris; gemelli; and obturator internus.

22. The surgical anatomy of the hip joint.

A. The hip joint is surrounded by a capsule which completely envelopes the femoral neck.

B. The artery of the ligamentum teres in the hip is the main blood supply of the adult femoral head.

C. The retinacular blood supply of the head of the femur may be disrupted by an intracapsular fracture of the femoral neck.

D. The superior gluteal nerve supplies the gluteus medius muscle.

E. The gluteus maximus is supplied by the sciatic nerve.

True:	C D
False:	A B E

The hip joint is surrounded by a capsule that extends posteriorly from the acetabulum rim to the mid-femoral neck, and anteriorly from the acetabulum rim to the intertrochanteric ridge. From the intertrochanteric ridge, some fibres of the joint capsule, known as retinacula, are reflected back up the neck to the head of the femur. These fibrous retinacula carry with them the retinacula blood vessels derived principally from the medial and lateral circumflex femoral vessels, the main blood supply to the adult head of the femur. Thus, disruption of the retinacula vessels by an intracapsular fractured neck of femur may render the head of the femur avascular. The superior gluteal nerve (L4, 5; S1) exits from the pelvis through the greater sciatic foramen above the piriformis muscle. It runs forward between the gluteus medius and minimus, supplying both, and ends by supplying the tensor fasciae latae. Damage to this nerve at operation will thus paralyse the abductors of the hip, precipitating the so-called Trendelenberg gait. The gluteus maximus is supplied by the inferior gluteal nerve. The sciatic nerve is related anteriorly to the gluteus maximus behind the hip and may be damaged at this site during operation by an injudiciously placed retractor. The sciatic nerve does not, however, supply gluteus maximus.

23. The direct lateral approach to the hip joint.

A. The transverse branch of the lateral circumflex artery is usually cut.

B. Requires careful dissection along the internervous plane between the superior gluteal nerve and the femoral nerve.

C. The lateral femoral cutaneous nerve is particularly at risk.

D. The fibres of gluteus medius are the first of the gluteals to be exposed.

E. The head of the femur is dislocated by internal rotation.

True:	A
False:	B C D E

The direct lateral approach (Hardinge approach) is the most commonly used approach for hemiarthroplasty of the hip joint. A longitudinal incision is made centred on the trochanter with a gentle posterior slope proximally. The superficial fascia and the fascia lata are cut to expose muscle. Gluteus maximus is retracted posteriorly and tensor fascia lata anteriorly to expose gluteus medius and vastus lateralis. The tendon of gluteus medius is then cut near its attachment to the greater trochanter and the same incision extended through vastus lateralis onto the anterior aspect of the femur. It is at this point that the transverse branch of the lateral circumflex artery is almost invariably cut and requires cautery. Detachment of gluteus medius and vastus lateralis exposes the capsule of the joint, which is usually cut in a T shape. Dislocation is achieved by adduction and external rotation. There is no true internervous plane in this approach. The femoral nerve is most at risk but primarily from positioning of retractors. The lateral cutaneous femoral nerve of the thigh is at risk in an anterior (Smith Petersen) approach to the hip where it lies in the internervous plane between sartorius (femoral nerve) and tensor fascia lata (superior gluteal nerve).

24. Posterior dislocation of the hip.

A. It classically occurs when the hip is in the flexed position.

B. It is a common injury.

C. The sciatic nerve may be permanently damaged.

D. The femur is usually medially rotated and flexed.

E. Avascular necrosis may occur.

True:	A C D E
False:	B

Posterior dislocation of the hip is a relatively uncommon injury and classically occurs when the hip is in the flexed position, e.g., car road-traffic-accidents (RTAs) with dashboard impact to the knees of front-seat passengers. In these patients, injury should also be expected to the knee joint, femur, and pelvis. Classically, with posterior dislocations, the leg appears short and the hip is held slightly flexed, adducted, and internally (medially) rotated. This deformity may reflect the position of the dislocated femoral head on the gluteal surface of the ilium. This leads to shortening of the extensors, abductors and external (lateral) rotators of the hip, and allows for unopposed action of the flexors, adductors and internal (medial) rotators of the hip. It should be emphasised, however, that the deformity of the hip seen in posterior dislocation may simply reflect the position of the femoral head once it has been displaced from the acetabulum. Two complications in particular are associated with posterior dislocation of the hip: sciatic nerve palsy (10–20%); and avascular necrosis of femoral head (10%). The sciatic nerve lies in close proximity to the capsule of the hip joint posteriorly and is, therefore, at risk in posterior dislocation. Fortunately, 75% of sciatic nerve palsies are incomplete, and >50% will recover completely. Prognosis is improved with early reduction of the hip, i.e., repositioning of the femoral head within the acetabulum. The sciatic nerve (L4, 5; S1–S3), is the largest nerve in the body and terminates by dividing into tibial and common peroneal nerves. Sciatic nerve palsy results in the following:

- Paralysis of knee flexion and all movement below the knee (resulting in foot drop).
- Complete sensory loss below the knee except for a small area on the medial side of the leg, which is supplied by the saphenous nerve.
- Loss of ankle jerk and plantar response, but the knee jerk is retained.

Avascular necrosis results from tearing of the joint capsule thereby disturbing the blood supply to the femoral head.

25. Intracapsular fractured neck of femur.

A. This is a relatively uncommon injury.

B. There is a high associated mortality.

C. Avascular necrosis of the femoral head is rare.

D. The hip is found to be medially rotated.

E. Sciatic nerve injury is a common complication.

True:	B
False:	A C D E

Fractured neck of femur (#NOF) is one of the commonest causes of emergency admission to orthopaedic wards, and occurs frequently in elderly and osteoporotic patients. These fractures can be classified most simply into extracapsular and intracapsular #NOFs. Both types are associated with considerable mortality (>30% at 6 months). This reflects the presence of associated disease and morbidity that may have caused the patient to fall in the first place. Intracapsular fractures account for 50% of #NOFs and more than 20% of these are complicated by avascular necrosis of the femoral head, due to disruption of the blood supply. Classically, the leg is found to be shortened and externally (laterally) rotated at the hip. Although hypotheses abound about which muscles cause this deformity, it is most likely that it arises simply as a result of gravity on a leg with a reflex reduction in muscular tone.

26. The bony structures of the knee joint.

A. The knee joint involves the articulation of the femur with the tibia and fibula.

B. The knee is a hinge joint, which undergoes flexion and extension only.

C. The patella articulates with the femur and the tibia.

D. The patella most commonly dislocates medially.

E. The tibia has a continuous articular surface with the femur.

All false.

The knee joint is a synovial joint between the condyles of the femur and the condyles of the tibia (the two tibial condyles are separated by an intercondylar ridge that attaches various ligamentous and cartilaginous structures). The fibula is not part of the joint and is not a weight-bearing bone. Although classified as a flexing and extending hinge joint, the knee can laterally and medially rotate when the joint is flexed and, in addition, there is some medial rotation of the femur in full extension. The patella is a sesamoid bone and articulates with the femur rather than covering the joint cavity. Due to a normal valgus position of the joint (i.e., there is an open angle on the lateral side of the knee), the patella is most commonly dislocated laterally. This injury is uncommon, due to the forward projection of the lateral condyle and the medial pull of vastus medialis on the patella.

27. The capsule, ligaments, and cartilages of the knee.

A. The lateral (fibular) collateral ligament is not part of the fibrous capsule.

B. The capsule completely seals the joint.

C. The anterior cruciate ligament (ACL) attaches to the medial condyle of the femur.

D. The medial meniscus (semilunar cartilage) is more commonly damaged than the lateral meniscus.

E. The lateral meniscus is smaller than the medial meniscus.

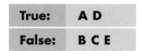

True:	**A D**
False:	**B C E**

The fibrous capsule of the knee joint is a cylinder of fibrous tissue between the femur and tibia, and includes the ligamentum patellae and the medial (tibial) collateral ligament but not the lateral (fibular) collateral ligament. It does not completely seal the knee joint and has two major openings: one for the suprapatella bursa in front; and one for the passage of the tendon of popliteus behind. The capsule is reinforced by the aponeuroses of the quadriceps and hamstrings, sartorius and the iliotibial tract. The ligaments of the knee joint can be divided into two groups, depending on their relationship to the capsule.

Extracapsular ligaments

- Ligamentum patellae – between the patella above and the tibial tuberosity below.

- Lateral collateral (fibular) ligament – between the lateral condyle of the femur and the head of the fibula below.

- Medial collateral ligament – between the medial condyle of the femur and the medial surface of the tibia below.

- Oblique popliteal ligament – this is a tendinous expansion of the semimembranosus muscle and strengthens the posterior aspect of the joint; its name refers to the oblique run of its fibres parallel to the popliteus muscle.

Intracapsular ligaments

- The two cruciate ligaments honour Scotland by forming a St. Andrew's cross within the joint, and join the condyles of the femur to the intercondylar ridge of the tibia. The ACL runs from the anterior part of the intercondylar ridge to the medial aspect of the lateral femoral condyle, while the posterior cruciate ligament (PCL) runs from the posterior part of the intercondylar ridge to the lateral aspect of the medial condyle of the tibia. The attachments of these ligaments can be remembered in various ways. One such way is to imagine that two little boxers are standing on the intercondylar ridge of the right knee, facing each other, i.e., one forwards (representing the PCL) and one backwards (representing the ACL). They both throw a right hook at each other and miss but hit the femoral condyles. The one at the front (ACL) hits the lateral femoral condyle while the one at the back (PCL) hits the medial femoral condyle. In the left knee, they would, of course, throw a left hook.

Of the two semilunar (half-moon shaped) cartilages, which are thought to act as shock absorbers between the femur and tibia, the medial meniscus is the largest. They are joined together anteriorly by a transverse ligament and they both attach to the intercondylar ridge anteriorly and posteriorly. There is an important difference in the attachments of the semilunar cartilages. The medial meniscus is closely attached to the joint capsule and, therefore, to the medial collateral ligament. The lateral meniscus has two extra ligaments attaching it to the femur (anterior and posterior meniscofemoral ligaments) and also attaches a slip of the tendon of the popliteus muscle which also separates it from the lateral aspect of the joint capsule. The end result of this arrangement is that the medial meniscus is more fixed in position than the lateral and is more commonly torn, e.g., in a lateral blow to the knee which stretches the attached medial collateral ligament.

28. The synovial membrane and the bursae of the knee joint.

A. The cruciate ligaments are intrasynovial.

B. The semimembranosus bursa frequently communicates with the synovial cavity.

C. The Infrapatella fold is filled by a fat pad.

D. The suprapatella bursa is attached to the vastus intermedialis muscle.

E. The prepatella bursa communicates with the synovial cavity.

True:	B C D
False:	A E

The synovial membrane lines the joint capsule, but passes in front of the cruciate ligaments which are, therefore, extrasynovial (but intracapsular). Anteriorly, the synovial membrane is separated from the ligamentum patellae by the infrapatella fat pad. The fold in the membrane that accommodates this fat pad is known as the infrapatella fold, and its free edges are known as the alar folds. There are at least 12 bursae associated with the knee joint; these can be divided conveniently into four groups of three bursae. The first group – bursae communicating with the knee – are important to know about because abnormal collections of fluid in the synovial cavity may show as swellings in these bursae, and infection of these bursae may spread into the joint with disastrous consequences (beware aspirating these bursae, as you may be responsible for introducing infection into the knee joint). The bursae around the knee joint can be summarised as follows.

Three bursae almost always communicating with the synovial cavity:

- Suprapatella (or quadriceps) bursa: extends three finger's-breadths above the patella beneath the quadriceps.
- Popliteus bursa: beneath popliteus tendon.
- Gastrocnemius bursa: deep to the medial head of gastrocnemius, this bursa often communicates with the bursa of semimembranosus which, therefore, also may communicate with the synovial cavity (hence why B above is true).

Three bursae related to the patella and ligamentum patellae:

- Prepatella bursa.
- Two infrapatella bursae: one superficial, one deep

Three hamstring bursae (includes semimembranosus bursa)

Three bursae around the collateral ligaments

29. Movements of the knee joint.

A. The knee joint may flex to 170°.

B. In full extension, the femur medially rotates on the tibia.

C. In full extension, the ACL is pulled tight.

D. Popliteus medially rotates the femur on the tibia.

E. The PCL is tight when the knee is in 90° flexion.

True:	B C
False:	A D E

The knee usually flexes little further than 135° due to limitation by contact with the soft tissues of the lower leg with the thigh. Just before the knee reaches full extension, the lateral condyle of the femur stops moving before the medial so that extension stops on the lateral side. As a result, the femur medially rotates on the tibia. In this position of slight hyperextension, all the ligaments (including the ACL and PCL) are taut, and the knee is said to be 'locked'. To 'unlock' the knee, the popliteus muscle contracts and laterally rotates the femur on the tibia (popliteus runs from the lateral surface of the lateral femoral condyle and lateral meniscus to the posterior surface of the tibia above the soleal line). In the position of 90° flexion, the ACL and PCL are slack and can be tested by the anterior drawer test (ACL prevents anterior movement of the tibia on the femur) and the posterior drawer test (PCL prevents posterior movement of the tibia on the femur).

30. The surgical anatomy of the knee joint.

A. The saphenous nerve and vein may be damaged in a medial approach to the knee.

B. The common peroneal nerve may be damaged in a lateral approach to the knee.

C. The principal blood supply of the knee is from the genicular branches of the femoral artery.

D. The innervation of the knee joint is exclusively by the femoral nerve.

E. The popliteal artery is the deepest of the NV structures in the popliteal fossa.

True:	A B E
False:	C D

The saphenous nerve and vein pass along the posteromedial border of the knee after emerging from behind sartorius. The saphenous nerve gives off an infrapatella branch to supply the anteromedial skin of the knee, and this should be protected in a medial parapatella approach to the knee. The common peroneal nerve emerges from behind biceps femoris to wind round the neck of the fibula. The common peroneal nerve may be damaged by a fracture of the neck of the fibula, producing a foot drop, as in the 'bumper bar injury' which may occur in a pedestrian hit by a motor vehicle. The genicular vessels which supply the knee are derived from the popliteal artery. The knee joint is supplied by branches of the femoral nerve, the TN, the common peroneal nerve and the obturator nerve.

31. The normal anatomy of the ankle joint.

A. Movements include inversion and eversion of the foot.

B. The deep deltoid ligament attaches the tibia to the calcaneus and navicular.

C. The syndesmosis is formed by a thickening in the interosseous membrane.

114

D. Three named nerves cross the ankle joint: sural nerve; saphenous nerve; and TN.

E. The sural nerve lies just medial to the Achilles tendon at the ankle.

All false.

The ankle joint is a synovial hinge joint between the tibia and fibula and the talus. Ankle movements are dorsiflexion (toes up) and plantar flexion (toes down): inversion and eversion of the foot take place at the subtalar joint between the talus and calcaneum. There are three groups of ligaments around the ankle: the deltoid ligaments; the lateral collateral ligamentous complex; and the syndesmosis. The deltoid ligament consists of a deep part, between the medial malleolus of the tibia and the talus, and a superficial part that is much weaker and stretches from the medial malleolus to the talus, calcaneus and navicular. The lateral collateral ligamentous complex consists of three bands: the anterior and posterior talofibular ligaments and the calcaneofibular ligament (the strongest of the three). The syndesmosis is perhaps the most significant ligamentous complex in maintaining normal alignment of the bones of the ankle joint. It consists of four parts: the anterior inferior talofibular ligament; the posterior inferior talofibular ligament; the inferior transverse tibiofibular ligament; and the interosseous ligament. Five named nerves cross the ankle joint and all provide sensation to different parts of the foot: the sural nerve (supplies the lateral border of the foot and little toe); the saphenous nerve (supplies the medial side of the foot down to the big toe); the TN (supplies the sole of the foot); the SPN (supplies the dorsal aspect of the foot except the first web space between the big toe and 2nd toe); and the DPN (supplies the first web space). It is essential to test the sensory integrity of these nerves in any ankle injury.

32.   The surgical anatomy of the ankle joint.

A. The ligamentous complex, which unites the distal tibia and fibula to form the ankle mortise, is referred to as the syndesmosis.

B. The horizontal articular surface of the ankle joint is referred to as the 'plafond'.

C. The supramalleolar portion of the ankle is referred to as the 'pilon' or 'pilon tibiale'.

D. From anterior to posterior, the structures immediately behind the medial malleolus are: the flexor hallucis longus tendon; the TN; the posterior tibial artery and vein; the FDL tendon; and the tibialis posterior tendon.

E. In the operative fixation of a fractured lateral malleolus, care must be taken to avoid damaging the saphenous nerve.

True:	A B C
False:	D E

Pilon tibiale refers to the French word for pestle, which the supramalleolar tibial flare is said to resemble. A 'pilon' fracture refers to a distal tibia/ankle fracture with supramalleolar involvement and damage to the plafond. The structures behind the medial malleolus from front to back are: tibialis posterior and flexor digitorum longus tendons, posterior tibial vein and artery and nerve, and most posteriorly the flexor hallucis longus tendon (remembered by the mnemonic 'Timothy Doth Vex All Nervous Housewives'). The sural nerve runs behind the distal fibula, and care should be taken to avoid it in fixing lateral malleolus fractures.

THE FOOT

33.   The bones of the foot.

A.   The cuboid bone is on the medial side of the foot.

B.   Peroneus longus attaches the 5th metatarsal.

C.   The talus, calcaneus and cuneiforms are part of the lateral arch.

D.   The 1st metatarsal articulates with the navicular.

E.   The talus is the most posterior bone.

All false.

Excluding sesamoid bones, there are 26 bones in the foot. There are the same number of metatarsals and phalanges as the corresponding metacarpals and phalanges in the hand. Posteriorly is the calcaneus with the talus sitting on top. These articulate anteriorly with the cuneiforms and the laterally placed cuboid. There are said to be three arches to the foot: two longitudinal and one transverse. The medial arch (calcaneus, talus, the three cuneiforms and medial three metatarsals) is said to be the strongest. The lateral arch is made up of the calcaneus, talus, cuboid, and the lateral two metatarsals. The transverse arch contains the cuneiforms, metatarsals and cuboid. These arches are incompletely understood, but they have become an accepted part of core anatomical knowledge. It suffices for the preclinical student to appreciate that the arches are supported by the shape of the bones, by the muscles and the ligaments (long and short plantar ligaments) and by the plantar aponeurosis. The end result is that the standing weight is taken on the calcaneus and metatarsal heads, and the arches help in giving spring to the foot in the take-off stage of walking.

34.   The muscles of the sole of the foot.

A.   Flexor digitorum accessorius inserts into FDL.

B.   Flexor digitorum brevis inserts into the middle phalanges of the lateral four toes.

C.   There are three dorsal interossei.

D.   The lumbricals arise from FDL.

E.   Flexor hallucis brevis lies deep to FDL.

All true.

The fine details of the musculature of the sole of the foot are important to the orthopaedic surgeon performing tendon transfers, correction of foot deformities, or operations such as Mitchell's osteotomy for bunions. It is useful for the non-specialist to appreciate that, in addition to long and short flexors of the toes, there are lumbricals and interossei that are organised in a similar fashion to their counterparts in the hand.

6. The Vertebral Column

TOPIC CHECK LIST

THE VERTEBRAL COLUMN

A.   All vertebrae have a body and a spinous process.

B.   The transverse process is attached to the body.

C.   The spinous process is formed by the junction of the pedicles posteriorly.

D.   The spinal cord lies posterior to the transverse processes.

E.   Marrow in the body of the vertebra is quiescent.

All false.

A typical vertebra consists of a body and a vertebral arch around a vertebral foramen. The vertebral arch consists of two pedicles from the back of the body, which attach to two laminae posteriorly. On each side of the vertebra, a transverse process attaches to the junction between the pedicle and the lamina (except L5 where the transverse process is joined to the vertebral body as well as the pedicle). The spinal cord lies in the vertebral canal formed by the vertebral arch, with the pedicles lateral and the transverse processes postero-lateral. The spinous process begins from the joint between the two laminae posteriorly. The first cervical vertebra has no body and no spinous process. Marrow in the vertebral body is a major site of blood cell production.

2.   The curvature of the vertebral column.

A.   There is only a single curve in the vertebral column of the fetus.

B.   In the adult there is a lumbar lordosis and cervical kyphosis.

C.   Secondary vertebral curves are predominantly due to the shape of the intervertebral discs.

D.   There are 33 free discrete vertebrae.

E.   There are eight cervical vertebrae.

True: A C

False: B D E

The fetal vertebral column has a single continuous anterior concavity. In the adult, two secondary curves appear (cervical and lumbar lordosis) due to changes in the shape of the intervertebral discs (and, in some cases, partly due to the shape of the vertebral bodies also). There are 33 vertebrae, but nine of them are fused in the sacrum and coccyx. There are seven cervical, 12 thoracic and five lumbar vertebrae. There are eight cervical spinal nerves.

3.   The cervical vertebrae.

A.   The 7th cervical vertebra is atypical.

B.   The axis articulates with the occipital bone.

C.   The foramen transversarium is in the transverse processes.

D. The vertebral artery passes through the transverse processes of C1–C7.

E. The dens is part of C2.

True:	A C E
False:	B D

The typical cervical vertebra has a small bifid spine and a foramen transversarium in the transverse processes. C1, C2 and C7 are atypical. C1 (atlas) has no body and is essentially a ring of bone that articulates with the occipital bone by two superior facets on each thick lateral mass; nodding and lateral flexion occurs at this joint. A four-part fracture of C1 in which the lateral masses of the ring are displaced laterally by axial loading, is referred to as a Jefferson fracture. C2 (axis) bears the dens (odontoid process, or peg) superiorly on its body. The dens represents the body of C1, and rotation of the skull occurs at the atlanto-axial joint. C7 (vertebra prominens) has the longest spinous process and is not bifid. Although the spinous process of C7 is the first easily palpable spine, the spine of T1 is the most prominent. The vertebral artery (from the subclavian) enters the foramen transversarium of C6 and passes through those of C5–C1 before entering the skull (through the foramen magnum). Vertebral veins pass through the foramen transversarium of C7.

4. The thoracic vertebrae.

A. All thoracic vertebrae have demi-facets for articulation with the rib heads.

B. The transverse processes articulate with the tubercles of the corresponding ribs.

C. The segmental spinal nerves come out below the corresponding vertebrae.

D. T5–T8 come into relation with the descending thoracic aorta.

E. The bodies decrease in size inferiorly.

True:	B C D
False:	A E

The 12 thoracic vertebrae have heart-shaped bodies which increase in size inferiorly. They are readily identified by the presence of a facet, or demi-facet, for the articulation with the heads of the ribs. T1 has, on each side, a facet for the first rib and a demifacet for the second rib. From T2 to T9, the bodies all have four demifacets: two superiorly, one on each side for the corresponding rib; and two inferiorly, one on each side for the rib below. T10, T11 and T12 all have two full facets, one on each side, for articulation with the corresponding rib. The transverse processes articulate with the tubercles of the corresponding ribs, except T11 and T12 because ribs 11 and 12 do not have tubercles and only articulate via their heads. An aneurysm of the thoracic aorta may erode the bodies of T5–T8 on their left anteriorly. The segmental spinal nerve C8 exits the spinal canal above T1, and thereafter the corresponding spinal nerve exits below the corresponding vertebra.

5. The lumbosacral vertebral column.

A. The articular surfaces of the superior articular facets of lumbosacral vertebrae face postero-laterally.

B. Lumbosacral vertebrae have no foramina in the transverse processes.

C. The laminae of the S5 (and sometimes S4) do not meet in the mid-line.

D. The spinal cord terminates in the sacral canal at S2.

E. There are 10 sacral foramina.

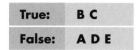

The articular surfaces of the superior articular facets face medially, and the inferior facets face laterally (c.f. postero-lateral and antero-medial in thoracic vertebrae). The sacral hiatus is formed by a defect in the laminae of S5 (and sometimes S4). The dura ends at S2, and the spinal cord terminates at L1/L2. There are four sacral foramina on each side, i.e., eight in total.

6. The joints and ligaments between vertebrae.

A. The facet joints are synovial joints.

B. The posterior ligament is not attached to the intervertebral discs.

C. C1 and C2 are joined by a fibrocartilage disc.

D. The dens is supported by only two named ligaments.

E. All joints between the bodies of the vertebrae are fibrocartilaginous.

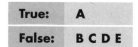

From C3 to the sacrum, the vertebrae are connected by the fibrocartilaginous joints between the bodies and synovial joints between the facets of the vertebral arches. The atlanto-occipital and atlanto-axial joints are synovial. In addition, there are small synovial joints at the sides of the intervertebral discs between the bodies of the lower cervical vertebrae. The bodies are supported from occiput to sacrum by continuous anterior and posterior longitudinal ligaments. The anterior longitudinal ligament is strong, wide, and firmly attached to both vertebral bodies and discs, whereas the posterior longitudinal ligament is weaker, narrower, and attached firmly only to the intervertebral discs. Superiorly, the longitudinal ligaments continue as the anterior and posterior atlanto-occipital membranes to attach to the foramen magnum. The vertebral arches are joined by three ligaments: the supraspinous ligament (between the tips of the spines); the interspinous ligaments (between the spines); and the ligamentum flavum (between laminae). The supraspinous and interspinous ligaments are thickened above C7 to form the ligamentum nuchae which attaches to the external occipital protruberance. The dens of the axis is held in place by three named sets of posterior ligaments: the apical ligament (median plane from tip of dens to foramen magnum); the alar ligaments (either side of the dens to the occipital condyles); and the cruciate ligament (a strong transverse part between the inner aspects of the lateral mass of the atlas, and a weak vertical part from the body of the axis to the foramen magnum). Damage to the transverse ligament with fracture through the dens, allows the skull and C1 to move forward on C2, and transection of the spinal cord results: this is referred to as the Hangman's fracture.

7. The intervertebral discs.

A. Contribute less than one-tenth of the length of the vertebral column.

B. Permit movement between adjacent vertebrae.

C. Are found between the bodies of all vertebrae.

D. Are attached to the anterior and posterior longitudinal ligaments.

E. The nucleus pulposus is situated anteriorly.

True:	B D
False:	A C E

The intervertebral discs contribute at least one-quarter of the length of the vertebral column and are absent between C1/C2 and sacrococcygeal vertebrae. They possess an outer anulus fibrosus consisting of fibrocartilage (concentric lamellae of collagen), and an inner nucleus fibrosus consisting of a cartilage/collagen/water semifluid gel. The discs are separated from the bodies of the vertebrae by hyaline cartilage. The discs act as shock absorbers and permit the vertebrae to move on one another. The nucleus pulposus lies slightly posteriorly and becomes less fluid with age. Herniation of the nucleus pulposus most commonly occurs in the lumbosacral and lower cervical regions (areas of mobile, on relatively immobile, vertebral column) and is usually posterior or lateral.

8. The blood supply of the vertebral column.

A. The vertebral arteries run in the spinal canal.

B. The vertebral arteries run the length of the vertebral column.

C. The vertebral venous plexus has many valves.

D. The vertebral venous plexus communicates with the intracranial venous sinuses.

E. The vertebral venous plexus does not communicate with the veins of the thorax.

True:	D
False:	A B C E

The vertebral artery (from subclavian) passes through the foramen transversarium of C6–C1. However, there are other arteries that also supply the cervical vertebrae: branches of the occipital artery; deep cervical artery (a branch of the costocervical trunk); and ascending cervical artery (a branch of the inferior thyroid). Thoracic vertebrae receive arterial blood from the posterior intercostal arteries. Lumbar vertebrae receive blood directly from the aorta via the lumbar arteries. The internal iliac artery gives branches to the sacrum. The valveless vertebral venous plexus has an external and internal part. There is free communication between both and with the segmental veins of thorax, abdomen and pelvis. The internal plexus (of Batson) lies within the vertebral canal outwith the dura, and communicates with the intracranial venous sinuses. This is an important route for the spread of malignancy between abdomen and brain.

9. The muscles of the vertebral column.

A. Splenius capitis is the uppermost muscle.

B. Semispinalis capitis lies deep to trapezius.

C. Erector spinae extends from the sacral region to the skull.

D. Posterior rami of all spinal nerves supply splenius capitis.

E. Quadratus lumborum attaches to the spinous processes.

True:	B C D
False:	A E

Erector spinae is the principle muscle of the vertebral column with which one should be familiar. It extends from the sacrum to the skull, filling the gap between the spinous processes and transverse processes. It is supplied by all posterior rami and extends the vertebral column. Superiorly it is known as semispinalis capitis and it lies deep to trapezius. Quadratus lumborum is part of the posterior abdominal wall and attaches to the 12th rib and the iliac crest.

7. Head and Neck

TOPIC CHECK LIST

REGIONS AND STRUCTURES OF THE NECK

1.   The fascial compartments of the neck.

A.   Platysma lies deep to the superficial fascia.

B.   The investing layer of deep fascia lies deep to trapezius.

C.   The axillary sheath is an extension of the prevertebral layer of deep fascia.

D.   Pretracheal fascia is attached to the fibrous pericardium inferiorly.

E.   The prevertebral fascia blends with the anterior longitudinal ligament of the spine at about C7.

F.   The retropharyngeal space extends from the skull to the mediastinum.

True:	C E F
False:	A B D

Knowledge of the fascial compartments of the neck is important clinically in appreciating the spread of infection and the lines of cleavage surgically. There is a superficial layer of fascia, which is a thin fatty membrane, enclosing platysma and the cutaneous nerves, vessels and lymphatics. The deep fascia is then split into investing, pretracheal, and prevertebral fascia and the carotid sheath. The investing fascia extends from the skull and mandible to the trunk, where it attaches to the manubrium, clavicle, and scapula. It can be envisaged by imagining a C-spine-immobilising collar on yourself. The investing fascia splits to enclose the trapezius, sternocleidomastoid and strap muscles, and the parotid and submandibular glands. The prevertebral fascia runs across the vertebrae and encloses the prevertebral muscles. It extends from the anterior longitudinal ligament of the spine at T3 inferiorly to the base of the skull superiorly and gives rise to the axillary sheaths which enclose the axillary vessels. This means that infection of the vertebral column may extend into the upper limb. In front of the prevertebral fascia is the pretracheal fascia, which encloses the thyroid, trachea, oesophagus and recurrent laryngeal nerves. This pretracheal fascia is important clinically for

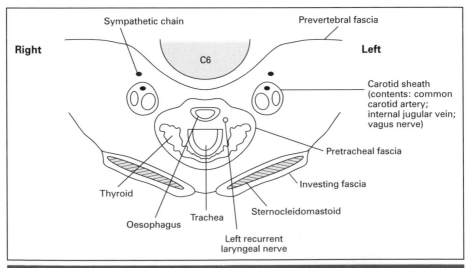

Fig. 51 The fascial layers of the neck and the relationships of structures in the neck at the level of the 6th cervical vertebra.

two reasons. Firstly, it is stronger anterior to the thyroid; therefore, if the thyroid enlarges pathologically, it is more likely to grow posteriorly and impinge upon the trachea. Secondly, between the pretracheal fascia and the prevertebral fascia is the retropharyngeal space, which extends from the skull to the mediastinum; pus may track up and down this space and air may enter the neck if the trachea ruptures. The pretracheal and prevertebral fasciae blend to form the separate structure known as the carotid sheath. The three layers of deep fascia are shown in *Figure 51*.

2. The carotid sheath.

A. Surrounds the carotid arteries, IJV and vagus nerve.

B. Is firmly attached to the sternocleidomastoid in front, and to the prevertebral fascia behind.

C. Is thinnest over the IJV.

D. Contains the ansa cervicalis.

E. Has the petrous part of the temporal bone as its upper attachment.

True: A C D E

False: B

The carotid sheath is made up of areolar tissue surrounding the carotids, the IJV and the vagus nerve. It is attached to the base of the skull at the margin of the carotid canal in the petrous part of the temporal bone, and continues down to the aortic arch. It is thin over the IJV, allowing dilatation for increased flow. The lower sheath is attached firmly to the posterior surface of the sternocleidomastoid muscle but posteriorly there is loose areolar tissue between the sheath and the prevertebral fascia; this is where the cervical sympathetic chain lies. The loose attachment allows spread of infection. The ansa cervicalis lies on the front of the IJV and is embedded in the anterior wall of the carotid sheath.

3. The anterior triangle of the neck.

A. It is bounded by sternocleidomastoid, trapezius and the clavicle.

B. It contains the axillary nerve.

C. It contains the submandibular gland and nodes.

D. It harbours the anterior strap muscles of the neck.

E. The hyoid bone lies at the level of C3.

True: C D E

False: A B

The anterior triangle of the neck is bounded by the sternocleidomastoid muscle, the angle of the jaw and the mid-line. The anterior triangle is further subdivided into the digastric, carotid and muscular triangles by the digastric and omohyoid muscles, respectively. The important contents of these triangles are as follows.

• Digastric triangle: submandibular gland and nodes, facial vessels, hypoglossal nerve.

• Muscular triangle: strap muscles of the neck, anterior jugular vein, jugular arch.

- Carotid triangle: carotid sheath and contents (IJV; common carotid artery, CC; Vagus), ansa cervicalis.

4. The posterior triangle of the neck.

A. Is bounded by sternocleidomastoid, trapezius and the clavicle.

B. Is traversed by the accessory nerve (XI).

C. Contains Virchow's node.

D. Contains the phrenic nerve.

E. Is where one would feel for the carotid pulse.

True:	A B C D
False:	E

The posterior triangle of the neck is important clinically because of the structures it contains. These include four important neural structures, as shown diagrammatically in *Figure 52*. The accessory nerve supplies trapezius and sternocleidomastoid, and damage to the nerve in the posterior triangle may cause a shoulder drop. The locations of the cervical plexus, the brachial plexus and

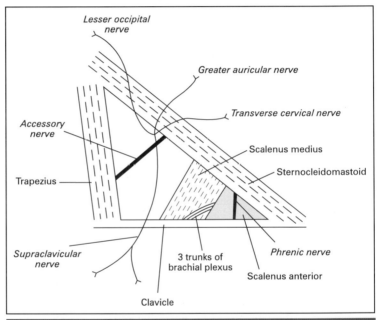

Fig. 52 Diagrammatic representation of the right posterior triangle of the neck, illustrating the main nerves situated in this region.

the phrenic nerve are important for the anaesthetist to know because all these nerves can be blocked in the posterior triangle. There are also important vascular structures in the posterior triangle, including the external jugular vein which crosses sternocleidomastoid to pierce the investing deep fascia in the lower medial corner of the triangle. Laceration of the external jugular vein here may result in an air embolus as tethering of the fascia to the vein prevents it from closing.

5. Relations of neck structures and the level C6.

A. The anterior and external jugular veins lie within the investing layer of fascia.

B. The carotid sheath encompasses the external carotid artery, IJV and vagus nerve.

C. The thyroid gland has the oesophagus as an immediate posterior relation.

D. The thyroid gland is encompassed in pretracheal fascia.

E. The recurrent laryngeal nerve is at risk of damage during thyroid surgery.

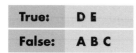

Figure 51 shows a cross-section of the neck at the level of C6. This important diagram alone should enable any student to remember the relations in the neck. From it, one can appreciate the important relations of the thyroid gland and also the many fascial planes in the head and neck. The close relationship of the recurrent and superior laryngeal nerves to the thyroid gland is foremost in the surgeon's mind, if he wishes to avoid litigation! The carotid sheath holds the common carotid, IJV and the vagus nerve. It is Important not to forget that, at the posterior margin of the carotid sheath, runs the sympathetic chain.

6. The thyroid gland.

A. The foramen lacerum in the tongue is a remnant of the thyroid gland's development.

B. The trachea lies anterior to the thyroid gland.

C. All blood supply to the thyroid gland is derived from the external carotid artery.

D. The inferior thyroid veins drain into the IJV.

E. The isthmus of the thyroid gland overlies the 2nd and 3rd tracheal rings.

True:	E
False:	A B C D

The foramen caecum at the junction of the middle and posterior thirds of the tongue is the remnant of the thyroid's descent into the neck; the foramen lacerum is a hole in the skull! If you refer to the cross-section through C6 (Figure 51) you will see clearly the relations of the thyroid gland. The trachea lies immediately behind the thyroid, within pretracheal fascia. The blood supply of the thyroid is rich and is a commonly asked question by examiners. The superior thyroid artery, one of the branches of external carotid in the neck, supplies the upper pole. The inferior thyroid artery comes from the thyrocervical trunk from the subclavian, and supplies the posterior aspect and lower pole of the gland. The much talked about, but of small significance, thyroid ima artery, when present (in up to 10% of the population), comes from the aorta or brachiocephalic trunk and supplies the isthmus. The veins follow the arteries. Superior thyroid and middle thyroid veins drain the upper pole and lateral aspects of the gland, respectively, and both drain into the IJV. The inferior thyroid vein drains the lower pole of the gland into the brachiocephalic veins. There is a rich anastomosis between the blood vessels supplying the gland. As a consequence, meticulous haemostasis is required when performing any thyroid surgery to avoid the complication of tracheal compression from an expanding haematoma. Finally, the isthmus of the gland, occasionally harbouring the pyramidal lobe, overlies the 2nd and 3rd tracheal rings.

7.   The external carotid artery.

A.   Arises at the level of the cricoid cartilage within the carotid sheath.

B.   Supplies the thyroid gland *via* the inferior thyroid artery.

C.   Is crossed by the glossopharyngeal and hypoglossal nerves.

D.   Supplies the palatine tonsil *via* the facial artery.

E.   Ends within the parotid gland, where it divides into its final two branches.

True:	C D E
False:	A B

The external carotid artery arises from the bifurcation of the CC at the level of C4, the upper level of the thyroid cartilage. It initially lies antero-medial to the internal carotid artery (ICA) but spirals around to lie lateral to it. It is crossed by the ansa cervicalis, the hypoglossal nerve and the facial nerve. The glossopharyngeal nerve and the pharyngeal branch of the vagus nerve cross between the external carotid artery and the ICA. The external carotid gives off six branches before terminating in the parotid gland as the maxillary and superficial temporal arteries. The six branch arteries are the superior thyroid, lingual, facial, occipital, posterior auricular, and ascending pharyngeal.

FACE AND SCALP

8.   Development of the face.

A.   The face is formed from the fusion of several processes around the stomadeum.

B.   Abnormalities of development are rare in the UK.

C.   Cleft lip is associated with syndactyly.

D.   Facial clefts are associated with spina bifida.

E.   Inclusional dermoids most commonly occur at the medial extremity of the upper eyebrow.

True:	A C D
False:	B E

The face develops from the fusion of frontonasal, maxillary and mandibular processes around the primitive mouth (stomadeum). As with all structures with a complex embryological origin, abnormalities are common and include facial cleft, cleft lip and cleft palate. Abnormalities of facial development are one of the commonest group of congenital abnormalities, with 1/600 children in the UK born with some form of cleft lip or palate. Anomalies of facial development are associated with a number of other congenital conditions, including syndactyly (fused digits) and spina bifida. Inclusional dermoids may form anywhere along the lines of fusion; the most common is at the lateral extremity of the upper eyebrow and is known as the external angular dermoid. This dermoid may connect to the dura through the skull.

9.   The cutaneous nerve supply of the face, scalp and neck.

A.   Skin is supplied entirely by branches of the trigeminal nerve (V) and of the cervical plexus.

B. The face is supplied entirely by the ophthalmic, maxillary and mandibular divisions of the trigeminal nerve.

C. The greater occipital nerve is a thin branch of the cervical plexus.

D. The cervical plexus is formed by the ventral rami of C1–C4.

E. The infratrochlear nerve is a branch of the maxillary branch of the trigeminal (V^b).

All false.

Skin of the head is mostly supplied by the trigeminal nerve and branches of the cervical plexus. However, there are two exceptions: Alderman's nerve, which is the cutaneous branch of the vagus (X), supplies the external auditory meatus and part of the auricle; and the greater occipital nerve, which supplies an area from the occipital protuberance as far as the vertex of the skull. The face is almost entirely supplied by the branches of V except for an area over the parotid and the angle of the jaw, which is supplied by the great auricular nerve. The greater occipital nerve is formed by the medial branch of the dorsal ramus of C2 and is the thickest cutaneous nerve of the body. The cervical plexus is formed by the ventral rami of C2–C4 (there is no cutaneous representation of C1). The infratrochlear nerve is a branch of the nasociliary nerve from the ophthalmic branch of the trigeminal (V^a).

10. The facial musculature.

A. All muscles are supplied by the facial nerve (VII).

B. Buccinator's most important function is in smiling.

C. Orbicularis oris is formed by several interdigitating muscles.

D. The eye is kept open by the action of occipitofrontalis, supplied by the temporal branch of the facial nerve.

E. Platysma is supplied by the cervical branch of the facial nerve.

True:	A C E
False:	**B D**

All muscles of facial expression are supplied by the facial nerve (VII) while the muscles of mastication (masseter and temporalis) are supplied by the motor root of the trigeminal (V). Buccinator's most important function is to prevent food accumulating in the vestibule of the mouth. The frontal belly of occipitofrontalis elevates the eyebrows; however, the eye is kept open by the action of levator palpebrae superioris supplied by the occulomotor nerve (III). It is easy to remember the nerves opening and closing the eye if you think of the Roman numeral III as three columns supporting the eyelid and the Arabic numeral 7 as a hook pulling the lid shut.

11. The arterial supply of the face and the scalp.

A. The superficial temporal artery is easily felt pulsating.

B. The transverse facial artery is a branch of the facial artery.

C. The facial artery lies deep to masseter.

D. The external carotid passes through the parotid gland.

E. The supraorbital artery is a branch of the external carotid.

True:	A D
False:	B C E

The superficial temporal pulse can be felt easily in front of the tragus. The transverse facial artery is a branch of the superficial temporal artery. The facial artery crosses the mandible just in front of masseter where it can be felt pulsating. The supraorbital and supratrochleal arteries are both branches of the internal carotid; all other scalp arteries are branches of the external carotid.

12. The venous drainage of the face and scalp.

A. The facial vein follows a tortuous course through the face.

B. Blood normally drains through emissary veins of the scalp into the intracranial venous sinuses.

C. The retromandibular vein drains into both the IJV and the external jugular vein.

D. The common facial vein drains into the IJV.

E. There is an anastomosis between the facial vein and the cavernous sinus *via* the orbit.

True:	C D E
False:	A B

It is the facial artery that follows a tortuous path (presumably reflecting the motility of the surrounding structures), whereas the facial vein has a much straighter course. Blood normally drains out *via* the emissary veins which, being valveless, are a route for the spread of infection into the skull. Similarly, infection can spread from the 'danger area' of the face *via* orbital anastomoses between the cavernous sinus and the facial vein.

13. The scalp.

A. The scalp is a loose structure with no bony attachments.

B. There are five named layers.

C. Occipitofrontalis attaches to the aponeurotic layer.

D. Blood vessels are found in the loose connective tissue layer.

E. Lymphatic drainage is to the deep cervical nodes.

True:	B C E
False:	A D

The scalp consists of five named layers: **S**kin; **C**onnective tissue; **A**poneurosis; **L**oose connective tissue; and **P**eriosteum (SCALP). The scalp is attached to the supraorbital margins anteriorly, the temporal fascia and zygomatic arches laterally, and the superior nuchal line posteriorly. The superficial three layers move as a unit and are collectively reflected as a flap in craniotomies. The connective tissue layer under the skin consists of tough fibrous septae with small fat lobules, and it is in this layer that the rich vasculature from the internal and external carotids runs. The aponeurotic layer contains the two bellies of occipitofrontalis.

MOUTH AND SALIVARY GLANDS

14. The parotid gland and duct.

A. The parotid gland overlies the posterior belly of digastric.

B. The ICA lies medial to the parotid duct.

C. A malignant tumour of the parotid can cause a facial nerve (VII) palsy.

D. The retromandibular vein lies deep to the parotid gland.

E. The parotid duct pierces buccinator opposite the 3rd upper molar tooth.

True:	A B C
False:	D E

The parotid gland is traversed by the facial nerve, retromandibular vein and external carotid artery. Tumours of the gland can, therefore, cause a facial nerve palsy. The parotid duct pierces buccinator opposite the 2nd upper molar tooth.

15. The submandibular region.

A. Mylohyoid and the anterior belly of digastric are 1st arch derivatives.

B. The posterior belly of digastric is supplied by the Vth cranial nerve.

C. The lingual artery lies deep to hyoglossus.

D. The hypoglossal nerve (XII) runs with the lingual artery.

E. The submandibular gland lies entirely superficial to mylohyoid.

True:	A C
False:	B D E

Underneath the superficial platysma muscle and the anterior and posterior bellies of the digastric, there are three muscles in the submandibular region, all of which attach to the hyoid bone. These are, from superficial to deep: mylohyoid; hyoglossus; and the middle constrictor of the pharynx. Because of the interesting embryology of this

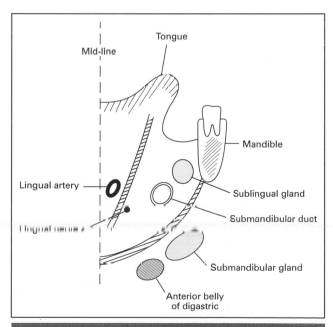

Fig. 53 Coronal section showing the general organisation of the submandibular glands in relation to the lingual artery and lingual nerve.

Labels: Mid-line; Tongue; Mandible; Lingual artery; Sublingual gland; Submandibular duct; Lingual nerve; Submandibular gland; Anterior belly of digastric

region, it is common for examiners to expect some understanding of how the innervation of the muscles can be explained. Mylohyoid, together with the anterior belly of digastric, is developed from the first branchial arch, and together the muscles are supplied by the Vth cranial nerve (through the mylohyoid nerve, which is a branch of the inferior alveolar nerve). The posterior belly of digastric is, however, a 2nd arch derivative and is, therefore, supplied by the facial nerve (VII). Hyoglossus, which inserts into the tongue, is supplied by the hypoglossal nerve (XII).

The two landmark muscles in the submandibular region are the mylohyoid and hyoglossus; an understanding of this region depends on knowing how the other structures lie in relation to these muscles. There are two salivary glands in the submandibular region: the submandibular gland and the sublingual gland. While both are superficial to hyoglossus, the latter lies entirely deep to mylohyoid, whereas the submandibular gland curves around the posterior margin of mylohyoid so that it is mainly more superficial. The lingual nerve and hypoglossal nerve both run with the submandibular duct of Wharton, deep to mylohyoid and superficial to hyoglossus. The lingual artery, however, runs deep to hyoglossus. The organisation of these structures is summarised in *Figure 53*.

16.	The muscles of mastication.

A. Temporalis and masseter close the mouth.

B. Side-to-side chewing movements are achieved by the alternate movement of the pterygoids.

C. The medial pterygoids are attached to the medial pterygoid plate.

D. All muscles of mastication are supplied by the Vth nerve.

E. The anterior belly of digastric and mylohyoid both act to depress the mandible and open the mouth.

True:	A B D E
False:	C

For the medical clinician, it will suffice to know that the motor branch of V innervates the muscles of mastication. Asking a patient to clench their teeth and then palpating masseter confirms the integrity of the motor branch of V. Anatomists and dentists demand a deeper knowledge of the muscles of mastication. Briefly, the medial and lateral pterygoids are responsible for the sideways movement of chewing, temporalis and masseter close the mouth, and the anterior belly of digastric and mylohyoid open the mouth. Both pterygoids attach to the lateral pterygoid plate of the skull but to the medial and lateral aspects, respectively.

17.	The temperomandibular joints.

A. Are simple ball-and-socket joints.

B. Allow for no lateral movement.

C. Have hyaline articular surfaces.

D. Move mainly symmetrically.

E. The axis of rotation in chewing lies on a transverse plane directly between the two joints.

All false.

The temperomandibular joints (TMJ) are the oldest synovial joints phylogenetically speaking (the lung-fish has only two synovial joints – the TMJs!). In man, they lie between the mandibular fossae of the temporal bones and the condyles of the mandible. They are both functionally divided into two separate joints by the presence of a fibrous intraarticular disc: the upper cavity allows for gliding movements and the lower for rotational movements. Opening and closing of the mouth involves rotation of the TMJ, with a transverse axis approximately half-way down the ramus of the mandible. Chewing, however, requires rotational movements that are predominantly asymmetrical.

18.   The infratemporal fossa.

A.   The lesser wing of the sphenoid forms part of the roof.

B.   The carotid sheath forms the posterior boundary.

C.   The infratemporal fossa contains the maxillary nerve.

D.   The infratemporal fossa contains the maxillary artery.

E.   The middle meningeal artery exits the fossa through the foramen spinosum.

True:	B D
False:	A C E

The infratemporal fossa is an important anatomical area because of its contents. It is best understood by holding a skull in the hand and identifying the boundaries. Essentially, the fossa has four bony boundaries: superiorly it lies under the temporal bone (hence its name), but the greater wing of the sphenoid also forms part of the roof; anteriorly lies the posterior surface of the maxilla; medially lies the lateral pterygoid plate; and laterally lies the ramus of the mandible. The fossa is, therefore, free inferiorly and bounded by the carotid sheath posteriorly. The important contents of the fossa are as follows: maxillary artery and its branches; mandibular nerve and its branches; medial and lateral pterygoid muscles, the otic ganglion; the chorda tympani; the pterygoid venous plexus; and the posterior superior alveolar nerve. The maxillary artery has 15 branches; the most important branches, however, are the middle meningeal artery, the sphenopalatine artery, the inferior alveolar artery, and the infraorbital artery. The middle meningeal artery passes into the skull through the foramen spinosum and it is this artery which is at risk of damage from a blow to the side of the head ('a punch in the temple'), leading to an extradural haemorrhage.

19.   The roof of the mouth.

A.   All muscles of the soft palate are innervated by the pharyngeal plexus.

B.   The pharyngeal plexus consists of fibres of the glossopharyngeal nerve (IX).

C.   Sensation to the roof of the mouth is provided by the facial nerve (VII).

D.   The hard palate consists of two palatine bones only, which meet in the mid-line.

E.   The blood supply to the roof of the mouth is through the maxillary artery.

True:	C E
False:	A B D

The roof of the mouth consists of the bony hard palate and the muscular soft palate. The hard palate is formed by the palatine processes of the maxillary bones anteriorly and the horizontal processes of the palatine bones posteriorly. Four muscles make up the soft palate: tensor palati; levator veli palati; palatoglossus; and palatopharyngeus. These muscles are all supplied by the pharyngeal plexus (fibres of XI), except for tensor palati, which is supplied by VII.

20. The tongue.

A. Genioglossus is an intrinsic muscle of the tongue.

B. Non-keratinised stratified squamous epithelium covers the entire surface of the tongue.

C. The vallate papillae receive innervation from the facial nerve (VII).

D. Taste from the posterior third of the tongue is supplied by the glossopharyngeal nerve (IX).

E. There is no communication of lymphatics across the mid-line of the tongue.

True:	D
False:	A B C E

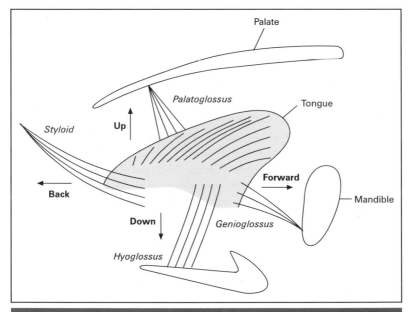

Fig. 54 Diagrammatic summary of the actions of the extrinsic muscles of the tongue.

The tongue is a mass of skeletal muscles covered by a mucous membrane and has a mid-line fibrous septum separating it into two halves. The surface of the tongue is covered by stratified squamous epithelium, which is keratinised in the anterior two-thirds and non-keratinised in the posterior third. At the boundary of the anterior two-thirds and posterior one-third is a structure known as the sulcus terminalis with large taste buds (known as vallate papillae) immediately anteriorly. The muscles of the tongue are divided into intrinsic and extrinsic muscles. The intrinsic muscles are organised into vertical, horizontal and transverse bundles; these fibres change the shape of the tongue. There are four extrinsic muscles of the tongue: genioglossus; hyoglossus; styloglossus; and palatoglossus. The direction in which the extrinsic muscles move the tongue can be understood by remembering their attachments (see Figure 54). Genioglossus protrudes the tongue and is the muscle that pulls the tongue forward to open the airway in the jaw-thrust manoeuvre. All the muscles of the tongue are supplied by the hypoglossal nerve (XII), except for palatoglossus which is supplied by XI *via* a pharyngeal branch of X. Innervation for common sensation and for special taste sensation is slightly more complex. The posterior third of the tongue and the vallate papillae receive fibres for common sensation and taste sensation from the glossopharyngeal nerve (IX). The anterior two-thirds of the tongue receives fibres for common sensation from V and for taste sensation from the chorda tympani (VII); both sets of fibres run in the lingual nerve. Although there is very little cross-anastomosis of lymphatics across the mid-line of the anterior two-thirds of the tongue, there is a rich cross-anastomosis in the posterior third where the fibrous raphe is very weak. Appreciation of this is important in understanding the spread of infection and metastasis from lingual tumours.

21. The teeth.

A. There are 20 deciduous (milk) teeth.

B. There are 20 permanent teeth.

C. The last tooth to erupt is the 3rd molar.

D. Nerve supply of the teeth is derived from fibres running in the maxillary nerve.

E. Maxillary sinusitis can result in toothache.

True:	A C D E
False:	B

There are four embryological arches in the mouth. Each arch produces two sets of teeth known as the deciduous (milk) teeth and the permanent teeth. The deciduous teeth erupt at about 6 months. There are 20 deciduous teeth, because in each arch there are two incisors, one canine, and two milk molars. The first permanent tooth is a molar and erupts at 6 years behind the milk molars. There are 32 permanent teeth in total, because in each arch there are two incisors, one canine, two premolars and three molars. The third molar is the last tooth to appear after the age of 18 years. The lower teeth are supplied by fibres of V^c through the inferior alveolar nerve. The upper teeth are innervated by fibres of V^b through the posterior, middle and anterior superior alveolar nerves. These nerves also provide sensation to the maxillary sinus; maxillary sinusitis often presents as toothache, due to referred pain.

EAR, NOSE AND THROAT

22. The nasal cavity.

A. The nasal septum is entirely cartilaginous.

B. The inferior concha is derived from the ethmoid bone.

C. The sphenoid sinus opens into the superior meatus.

D. Epistaxis can be controlled by ligating the maxillary artery.

E. General sensation from the nasal cavity is carried by the trigeminal nerve (V).

True:	D E
False:	A B C

There are two nasal cavities separated by a median nasal septum that consists of septal cartilage and two bony parts: the vomer and the perpendicular plate of the ethmoid bone. Each cavity is approximately 5 cm high and 7 cm long extending from the nares anteriorly to the choanae posteriorly. The lateral walls of each cavity are made up mostly from the maxilla, but the lacrimal, ethmoid and palatine bone also contribute. The ethmoid bone gives rise to the two upper protrusions from the lateral walls known as the superior and middle conchae. The inferior choncha is a separate bone. The space above the superior concha is known as the sphenoethmoidal recess. The spaces below the conchae are known as the superior, middle and inferior meatus. The structures draining into each space are summarised below.

Sphenoethmoidal recess

- Sphenoidal sinus

Superior meatus

- Posterior ethmoidal sinus

Middle meatus

- Frontal sinus
- Maxillary sinus
- Anterior and middle ethmoidal sinus

Inferior meatus

- Nasolacrimal duct

The main arterial supply to the septum and lateral walls is the sphenopalatine artery, a branch of the maxillary artery which can be ligated in the event of uncontrollable epistaxis. The olfactory nerve (I) supplies special sensation, but common sensation from the nasal mucosa is carried by branches of the trigeminal nerve (V).

---

23. The pharynx.

A. The posterior pillar of the oropharynx is formed by the palatoglossus muscle.

B. Stylopharyngeus is supplied by the recurrent laryngeal nerve.

C. The constrictor muscles are enclosed in the same fascia as buccinator.

D. The Eustachian tube enters the pharynx just below the soft palate.

E. The palatine tonsils receive arterial blood from the facial artery.

True:	C E
False:	A B D

The pharynx is a musculofascial tube which extends from the base of the skull to the oesophagus, and acts as a common opening to the respiratory and alimentary tracts. Its shape is often compared to a ships funnel, and it is divided into three parts: the nasopharynx; the oropharynx; and the laryngopharynx. *Figure 55* shows diagrammatically the three parts and their contents. The nasopharynx lies above the soft palate and extends to the choanae at the posterior limit of the nasal cavities. The nasopharynx contains the nasopharyngeal tonsils (adenoids) in children and the opening to the Eustachian tube, which communicates with the middle ear. The oropharynx extends from the uvula and the anterior pillars to the tip of the epiglottis. The anterior pillars are formed by palatoglossus, and the posterior pillars by palatopharyngeus. The region between the two pillars contains the palatine tonsils, which receive blood from a tonsilar branch of the facial artery. The laryngopharynx extends from the tip of the epiglottis to the oesophagus, at the level of C6. The pharynx walls consist of a mucosa (ciliated columnar epithelium in the nasopharynx and stratified squamous epithelium in the oro- and laryngopharynx), a submucosa, and the muscular layer. The muscle layer consists of three horizontal constrictors, which are telescoped together and are known as superior, middle and inferior constrictors. The inferior constrictor is divided into two parts known as thyropharyngeus and cricopharyngeus. Pharyngeal mucosa may protrude between these two muscles through a gap known as Killian's dehiscence, and form a pharyngeal pouch where food may get trapped. All constrictor muscles are covered by an areolar sheath known as the buccopharyngeal fascia because it also covers the buccinator muscles. There are also three longitudinal muscles of the pharynx known as palatopharyngeus, stylopharyngeus and salpingopharyngeus. All muscles of the pharynx are innervated by the pharyngeal plexus (IX and X), except for stylopharyngeus (IX alone) and cricopharyngeus (external laryngeal nerve).

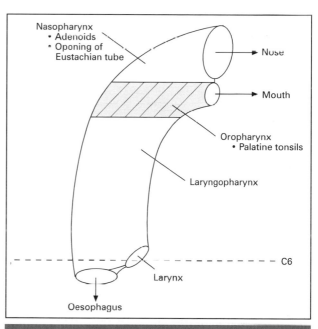

Fig. 55 Diagrammatic representation of the pharynx.

24. The larynx.

A. The primary function of the larynx is speech.

B. The hyoid bone lies at the level of C3.

C. The cricoid is a VIth arch derivative.

D. The posterior cricoarytenoid muscles are the only muscles opening the vocal cords.

E. The piriform fossa is part of the vestibule of the larynx.

F. The vocal cords are part of the cricovocal membrane (conus elasticus).

G. All the intrinsic muscles of the larynx are supplied by the recurrent laryngeal nerve.

True:	B C D F
False:	A E G

The larynx is a framework of articulating cartilages linked by ligaments. These cartilages move in relation to one another by the action of laryngeal muscles. The primary function of the larynx is to protect the lower respiratory tract from inhalation of foreign bodies. It also has a secondary function of controlling the pitch of speech in humans (phonation is also a product of the pressure of air through the larynx and the shape of the resonating air chambers above the glottis, i.e., pharynx, nose and mouth). There are four main laryngeal cartilages: the thyroid cartilage; the arytenoid cartilage; the cricoid cartilage; and the epiglottis. There are also the less important, miniscule corniculate and cuneiform cartilages. It is important to remember the vertebral levels of the thyroid and cricoid laryngeal cartilages, and it is a useful *aide memoire* that some of these levels correspond to their embryological arches. The top of the thyroid cartilage lies at the level of C4 and is a IVth arch derivative. The cricoid lies at the level of C6 and is a VIth arch derivative. There are various ligaments linking the laryngeal cartilages, but the one with which it is most important to be familiar is the cricovocal membrane (the conus elasticus), which extends upwards like a tent from the cricoid cartilage to the thyroid cartilage. Anteriorly, this is thickened to form the cricothyroid ligament, which is pierced in an emergency (if the upper airways are blocked) by the procedure known as cricothyroidotomy. Superiorly, the conus elasticus folds to form the vocal ligaments (vocal cords). The muscles of the larynx are classified into extrinsic muscles, which move the larynx as a whole, and the intrinsic muscles, which act on the vocal cords. There are basically three functions fulfilled by the intrinsic muscles: opening the cords (the posterior cricoarytenoids only!); closing the larynx during deglutition (lateral cricoarytenoids); and altering the tension of the cords during speech (the thyroarytenoids reduce the tension, and the cricothyroids increase the tension). All the intrinsic muscles, except cricothyroid, are supplied by the recurrent laryngeal nerve; cricothyroid is supplied by the superior laryngeal nerve.

25. The middle ear.

A. Lies in the temporal bone.

B. The incus is attached to the tympanic membrane.

C. Tensor tympani muscle is supplied by the mandibular nerve.

D. The auditory tube opens into the medial wall.

E. The base of stapes occludes the fenestra vestibuli.

True:	A C E
False:	B D

The tympanic membrane lies in the lateral wall; the handle of the malleus is attached to the tympanic membrane. The posterior wall contains the mastoid antrum and the facial nerve. The medial wall separates the middle ear from the vestibule and cochlea. The anterior wall contains the auditory tube and carotid canal. The roof is formed by a thin plate of bone (tegmen tympani) that separates the middle ear from the middle cranial fossa. The floor is also formed by a thin plate of bone and separates the jugular bulb from the middle ear. The incus is attached to the malleus; the stapes is attached to the incus. Two muscles, tensor tympani and stapedius muscle, damp down the movements of the ossicles. Tensor tympani is attached to the handle of the malleus. Stapedius muscle is attached to the body of the stapes and is supplied by the facial nerve.

26.   The lymphatic drainage of the head and neck.

A.   The superficial cervical nodes always drain into the deep cervical chain.

B.   Superficial tissues of the head always drain into the 'horizontal circle' of nodes.

C.   Retropharyngeal nodes drain directly into the thoracic duct.

D.   The deep cervical nodes lie along the external jugular vein.

E.   All nodes eventually drain into the thoracic duct.

True:	A
False:	**B C D E**

All head and neck structures drain, directly or indirectly, through the deep cervical nodes. Lymph then drains into the thoracic duct on the left, or the right lymphatic duct on the right. Superficial tissues drain mainly to the 'horizontal circle' of nodes (submental, submandibular, periauricular, mastoid, and suboccipital) and then to the deep cervical nodes. However, some lymph vessels will drain directly to the deep cervical nodes.

INTRACRANIAL REGION AND ORBIT

27.   The intracranial fossae.

A.   The crista gallae is part of the frontal bones.

B.   The motor root of V passes through the foramen rotundum.

C.   Cranial nerves III, IV, V and VI pass through the inferior orbital fissure.

D.   The cerebellum lies above the tentorium cerebelli in the posterior cranial fossae.

E.   The jugular foramen is in the middle cranial fossa.

All false.

The inner base of the skull can be divided into anterior, middle and posterior cranial fossae. It is important to have an appreciation of the boundaries of these fossae and of the gross structures found in each, and to know the main NV structures passing through the foramina. This is best done whilst holding an open skull. The anterior cranial fossa is formed by the frontal bones anteriorly and is bounded posteriorly by the anterior clinoid processes of the sphenoid bone and the lesser wings of the sphenoid. In the mid-line of the anterior part of the anterior cranial fossa is the cribriform plate of the ethmoid bone and the mid-line crista gallae (Cock's comb). The middle cranial fossa is formed by the petrous part of the temporal bones, and the body and greater wings of the sphenoid bone. It extends from the posterior border of the anterior cranial fossa in front, to the crest of the petrous part of the temporal bone behind. The posterior cranial fossa extends from here to the occipital bone at the back of the skull. The contents of each fossa and the NV structures passing through the skull in each fossa are summarised below.

Anterior cranial fossa

*   Frontal lobes.

*   Olfactory tract.

*   Olfactory bulb on the cribriform plate.

- Olfactory fibres pass through the cribriform plate.
- The foramen caecum transmits emissary veins from the nasal cavity to the superior sagittal sinus.

Middle cranial fossa

- Temporal lobes.
- ICA.
- Middle meningeal artery.
- Carvernous sinus.
- Hypothalamus and pituitary.
- Trigeminal ganglion.
- The superior orbital fissure transmits III, IV, V^a, and VI.
- The foramen rotundum transmits V^b.
- The FO transmits the motor root of V and the accessory meningeal artery.
- The foramen spinosum transmits the middle meningeal artery.

Posterior cranial fossa

- Hindbrain.
- Cerebellum (below the tentorium cerebelli).
- The foramen magnum transmits the lower medulla/spinal cord, the vertebral arteries, the vertebral venous plexus, and the spinal roots of IX.
- The hypoglossal canal transmits XII.
- The jugular foramen transmits IX, X, and XII.
- The internal acoustic meatus transmits VII and VIII.

28. Cranial meninges and intracranial venous sinuses.

A. Pia is the innermost of the meninges.

B. The cranial blood sinuses are valveless.

C. The intracranial venous sinuses are formed by duramater.

D. The superior ophthalmic veins connect the cavernous sinuses to the facial vein.

E. Cranial nerves III, IV, V^a, and V^b all pass through the cavernous sinuses.

F. Meningeal arteries lie in the subarachnoid space.

True:	A B C D
False:	E F

There are three layers of cranial meninges that are named, from outwards in: dura, arachnoid, and pia. The valveless intracranial blood sinuses are formed by the dura. The venous sinuses are the venous drainage of the brain and are also involved in the circulation of cerebrospinal fluid (CSF). The cavernous sinuses are connected to the facial veins *via* the superior ophthalmic veins; this is an important route for the spread of infection from the face and can result in cavernous sinus thrombosis. Cranial nerve VI and the ICA traverse the cavernous sinus; thrombosis here can result in a VIth nerve palsy and conjunctival oedema. Arterial branches of the circle of Willis, which supply the brain, run in the subarachnoid space. Meningeal arteries run outside the dura and their rupture can result in extradural haemorrhage.

29. The orbit.

A. The greater and lesser wings of the sphenoid bone both form part of the orbit wall.

B. The ethmoid bone forms part of the lateral wall.

C. All muscles moving the eye originate from a fibrous ring at the back of the orbit.

D. Superior oblique moves the eye downwards and outwards.

E. Superior rectus moves the eye directly upwards.

F. Inferior oblique is supplied by cranial nerve IV.

G. Lateral rectus is supplied by cranial nerve VI.

H. The ophthalmic artery is derived from the ICA.

True:	A D G H
False:	B C E F

The walls of the orbit are formed by the frontal bone superiorly, the maxilla inferiorly and the zygomatic bone laterally. Medially are the lacrimal and ethmoid bones. Both wings of the sphenoid bone form part of the posterior wall of the orbit. All the muscles moving the eye, except inferior oblique, originate from a fibrous ring at the back of the eye. The innervation of these muscles can be remembered using the 'formula' LR_6SO_4: lateral rectus is supplied by VI; superior oblique is supplied by IV; all the others are supplied by III.

8. Neuroanatomy

TOPIC CHECK LIST

NEUROANATOMY

A. The lateral corticospinal tract contains crossed motor fibres.

B. Pain and temperature sensation is carried in the dorsal columns of the spinal cord.

C. Joint position sense in the thumb is carried through the cuneate tract.

D. Axons travelling in the spinothalamic tract cross over in the medulla.

E. The spinocerebellar tracts carry information involved in the control of movement and posture.

True:	A C E
False:	**B D**

The long tracts of the spinal cord are either sensory or motor. Ascending pathways are sensory and the descending pathways are motor. The main sensory pathways are as follows.

Spinothalamic tract

• This carries pain and temperature fibres. Afferent fibres enter the posterior horn of the spinal cord, synapse and immediately cross over (decussate) to the contralateral side. They then ascend in the spinothalamic tract, which lies in the anterior/lateral part of the cord.

Gracile and cuneate tracts

• These carry the fibres for light touch, vibration and proprioception, and form the dorsal columns of the spinal cord. The gracile tract carries fibres from the lower limb, whereas the cuneate tract carries fibres from the upper limb and so is found only in the upper part of the spinal cord. Axons carrying these modalities of sensation enter the posterior horn of the spinal cord ascending on the ipsilateral side without synapsing. These fibres synapse in the medulla (in the gracile and cuneate nuclei), cross over and travel in the medial lemniscus.

Spinocerebellar tracts

• These carry information from the periphery to the cerebellum. They lie in the lateral part of the spinal cord and carry both crossed and uncrossed fibres. They carry information involved in the control of movement and posture.

The corticospinal tract is the main descending pathway, carrying motor fibres to the periphery. These descending fibres cross over in the medulla and travel in the lateral corticospinal tract. Uncrossed fibres also descend in the much smaller anterior corticospinal tract.

A right-sided spinal cord hemisection (Brown-Séquard syndrome) at T1 may result in the following.

A. A Horner's syndrome on the right.

B. Loss of pain and temperature sensation in the right leg.

C. Wasting of the 1st dorsal interosseous muscle of the right hand.

D. Loss of light touch and proprioception of the left hallux.

E. Weakness in the right leg.

True:	A C E
False:	B D

The Brown-Séquard syndrome is a hemisection of the spinal cord. A lesion at T1 will affect both ascending and descending pathways. There will be an ipsilateral monoplegia, and loss of light touch and proprioception. In addition, there is a contralateral loss of pain and light touch sensation. Motor fibres supplying the small muscles of the hand originate at T1 and so there will be wasting of these muscles. In addition, the patient may present with a Horner's syndrome on the same side. Sympathetic outflow is from T1 to L2. A lesion at T1 will prevent sympathetic information travelling up to the sympathetic cervical ganglia and so may lead to the features of Horner's syndrome.

3. Brainstem ascending and descending pathways.

A. The ascending spinothalamic tract continues as the medial lemniscus.

B. Decussation of the pyramids occurs in the medulla.

C. The fasciculus gracilis carries proprioceptive information from the upper limbs.

D. Damage to the medullary pyramids prior to decussation leads to an ipsilateral weakness of muscles of facial expression and a contralateral hemiplegia.

E. Fibres travelling from pons to cerebellum pass through the middle cerebellar peduncle.

True:	B E
False:	A C D

Descending motor fibres are carried in the cerebral peduncles, travelling down in the pyramids. The pyramids decussate in the medulla. Damage here prior to decussation leads to a contralateral hemiplegia. The muscles of facial expression are spared because the facial motor nucleus is contained in the pons. The gracile and cuneate tracts carry light touch and proprioceptive information from the lower and upper limbs, respectively, and continue their ascent as the medial lemniscus. The spinothalamic tract ascends as the spinal lemniscus. The brainstem also has connections with the cerebellum. This occurs through the superior, middle and inferior cerebellar peduncles to the midbrain, pons and medulla, respectively.

4. Brainstem structures.

A. The 4th ventricle is found at the level of the closed medulla.

B. The inferior colliculus sends afferents to the lateral geniculate nucleus (LGN).

C. The superior colliculus mediates smooth pursuit eye movements.

D. The pretectal nucleus mediates the pupillary accommodation reflex.

E. The periaqueductal grey matter is involved in pain perception.

True:	C E
False:	A B D

The 4th ventricle is found at the level of the open medulla. The inferior colliculus, in the midbrain, is involved in the auditory system, so sends efferents to the medial geniculate nucleus. The superior colliculus is involved in the visual system and mediates the body's response to light/movement and the smooth pursuit visual system. The pretectal nucleus is involved in the pupillary light reflex. The accommodation reflex is mediated through the supplementary visual cortex in the occipital lobe. The periaqueductal grey matter is an area of myelinated axons that is found around the cerebral aqueduct. It is involved with the perception of pain, and has higher cortical connections.

5. Features of a complete IIIrd nerve palsy.

A. Ptosis.

B. Constricted pupil.

C. Ipsilateral loss of sweating.

D. Laterally deviated eye.

E. Loss of function of the superior oblique muscle.

True:	A D
False:	B C E

The oculomotor nerve carries both motor and autonomic fibres. It is motor to all the muscles of eye movement, except the lateral rectus and superior oblique muscles. In addition, it carries sympathetic fibres to levator palpebrae superioris. Parasympathetic fibres originate from the Edinger-Westphal nucleus and are carried by the IIIrd nerve, synapsing at the ciliary ganglion. Postganglionic parasympathetic fibres are responsible for pupillary constriction. A complete lesion of the IIIrd nerve may occur in intracranial bleeds, leading to herniation of the uncus of the temporal lobe. This compresses the oculomotor nerve, leading to the characteristic features of a ptosis, dilated pupil and a laterally deviated eye. It is important to differentiate between a IIIrd nerve palsy and a Horner's syndrome (damage to cervical sympathetic chain). This latter condition presents with a ptosis, constricted pupil and loss of sweating on the affected side.

6. The VIIth cranial nerve.

A. Carries preganglionic parasympathetic fibres to the lacrimal gland.

B. Supplies taste to the anterior two-thirds of the tongue.

C. Is involved in mediation of the corneal reflex.

D. An upper motor neuron lesion causes paralysis of orbicularis oculi.

E. The nucleus lies in the pons.

True:	A B C E
False:	D

The facial nerve is a sensory and motor nerve. The motor nucleus is contained within the pons. These efferent axons run with the nervus intermedius into the internal auditory meatus, through the middle ear, and out of the intracranial region through the stylomastoid foramen. The main supply is to the muscles of facial expression. Due to bilateral innervation, from both motor cortices, of the muscles of the upper half of the face, an upper motor neuron lesion affecting the facial nerve will spare the muscles around the eye. A lower motor neuron lesion will affect all the muscles of facial expression on that side of the face. The motor nucleus of the facial nerve also plays a role in the efferent loop of the corneal reflex. Stimulation of the cornea sends afferents through the Vth nerve to the facial motor nucleus; efferents *via* the facial nerve cause stimulation of orbicularis oculi and thus blinking to occur. The sensory root (nervus intermedius) carries special sensory fibres receiving taste information from the anterior two-thirds of the tongue. These fibres synapse in the geniculate ganglion before terminating in the solitary nucleus of the medulla. The nervus intermedius also carries parasympathetic fibres supplying the lacrimal gland, as well as the submandibular and sublingual salivary glands. These fibres are sent out from the superior salivatory nucleus, with the preganglionic fibres for the lacrimal glands synapsing in the pterygopalatine ganglion, and the preganglionic fibres for the salivary glands synapsing in the submandibular ganglion.

7. General organisation of the brain.

A. The primary motor cortex is located in the frontal lobe.

B. Wernicke's area is in the parietal lobe.

C. The somatosensory cortex is found in the precentral gyrus.

D. Broca's area is in the temporal lobe.

E. The primary auditory cortex is found in the superior temporal gyrus.

True:	A E
False:	B C D

The brain can be divided into the two hemispheres by the longitudinal fissure. Each hemisphere can be divided into different lobes by folds of the brain – gyri and sulci. The frontal lobe is separated from the parietal lobe by the central sulcus. The precentral gyrus, contained in the frontal lobe, contains the primary motor cortex. The postcentral gyrus, in the parietal lobe, contains the somatosensory cortex. The temporal lobe is separated from the parietal lobe by the lateral fissure. The auditory cortex is contained here in the superior temporal gyrus. The occipital lobe contains the primary visual cortex. The major speech and language centres of the brain are contained in the left hemisphere of the brain. Broca's area in the frontal lobe is responsible for speech. Wernicke's area in the temporal lobe is involved in the understanding of speech.

8. The cerebellum.

A. Is connected to the pons *via* the middle cerebellar peduncle.

B. Lies in the posterior cranial fossa.

C. Is supplied by branches of the posterior cerebral artery.

D. The anterior and posterior lobes are separated by the horizontal fissure.

E. Damage to the dentate nucleus affects equilibrium and balance.

True:	A B
False:	C D E

The cerebellum is a component of the hindbrain, lying in the posterior cranial fossa of the brain, below the tentorium cerebelli. It coordinates movement and is involved in balance. It contains connections to the different parts of the brainstem. The cerebellum is connected to the midbrain, pons and medulla *via* the superior, middle and inferior cerebellar peduncles, respectively. The cerebellum is made up of two hemispheres linked by the mid-line vermis. It is thrown into folds, which separate the cerebellum into different lobes. These lobes are the anterior and posterior lobes, which are separated by the primary fissure, and the flocculonodular lobe. Within the cerebellar white matter are contained a number of nuclei. The largest of these is the dentate nucleus, which is concerned with coordination of movement. Equilibrium and balance is controlled through the flocculonodular lobe.

9. The primary visual cortex.

A.   Lies completely below the calcarine sulcus.

B.   Its anterior one-third represents the macula.

C.   Receives projections from the LGN.

D.   Is supplied by the middle cerebral artery.

E.   Mediates the pupillary light reflex.

True:	C D
False:	A B E

The primary visual cortex is situated in the occipital lobe of the brain. It lies on the medial surface of the cerebral hemisphere, on either side of the calcarine sulcus. It receives fibres through the optic radiation, which project from the LGN. There is point-to-point mapping of retinal projections onto the visual cortex. The peripheral visual field is represented in the anterior two-thirds of the cortex, with the macula occupying the posterior one-third. Blood supply is mainly through the posterior cerebral artery, but the macula has a dual blood supply through both the posterior and middle cerebral arteries. Pupillary light reflexes are mediated through the pretectal nuclei in the midbrain.

10. The central visual pathways.

A.   All fibres in the optic tract synapse in the LGN.

B.   Damage to the optic chiasma will characteristically produce a bitemporal hemianopia.

C.   A lesion of the optic radiation in Meyer's loop causes a lower quadrantanopia.

D.   The optic radiation passes through the internal capsule.

E.   A middle cerebral artery infarct will produce a homonymous hemianopia with macular sparing.

True:	B D
False:	A C E

Light hitting the back of the eye is processed by the retina. Axons travel through the optic nerve to the optic chiasma, where there is crossover of fibres from the temporal visual field (or nasal hemiretina). The optic tracts, containing the ipsilateral temporal hemiretina and contralateral nasal hemiretina, extend backwards around the cerebral peduncle. The majority of fibres synapse in the LGN. A smaller number bypass the LGN and pass in the superior brachium to the midbrain, with terminations in the pretectal nucleus and superior colliculus. From the LGN, fibres sweep back in the optic radiation. They run in the retrolenticular part of the internal capsule. Those fibres that represent the upper part of the visual field are mapped onto the visual cortex below the calcarine sulcus. This part of the optic radiation initially sweeps into the temporal lobe, forming a loop known as Meyer's loop. The part of the optic radiation that projects to the visual cortex above the calcarine sulcus travels in the parietal lobe.

11. The basal ganglia.

A. The locus coerulus is part of the basal ganglia.

B. The anterior limb of the internal capsule separates the caudate from the putamen.

C. The claustrum lies lateral to the lentiform nucleus.

D. The head of the caudate is closely related to the lateral ventricle.

E. The globus pallidus is supplied by the anterior choroidal artery.

F. The posterior limb of the internal capsule separates the caudate nucleus from the thalamus.

True:	B C D E
False:	A F

Functionally, the basal ganglia are made up of the corpus striatum, subthalamic nucleus and substantia nigra. The corpus striatum is composed of the caudate nucleus, putamen and globus pallidus (these latter two form the lentiform nucleus). The caudate nucleus consists of a head and a tail. The head lies lateral to the anterior horn of the lateral ventricle. The anterior limb of the internal capsule separates it from the putamen. The putamen is separated from the thalamus by the posterior limb of the internal capsule. Lying lateral to the lentiform nucleus is the claustrum, external capsule and insula. Blood supply is derived from branches of the middle cerebral, anterior cerebral and anterior choroidal arteries. The globus pallidus is supplied by the anterior choroidal artery.

12. The internal capsule.

A. Corticospinal tract fibres are carried in the anterior limb.

B. The internal capsule separates the caudate and putamen.

C. Spinothalamic tract fibres run in the posterior limb.

D. The internal capsule is supplied by the anterior choroidal artery.

E. The internal capsule is supplied by the middle cerebral artery.

True:	B C D E
False:	A

The internal capsule is a mass of projection fibres; it lies with the lentiform nucleus laterally, and the head of the caudate and diencephalons medially. The different parts can be described in relation to the lentiform, i.e., as supralenticular, sublenticular or retrolenticular. The internal capsule is distorted in shape, forming an anterior limb, genu and posterior limb. The anterior limb contains connections between the thalamus and premotor cortex, as well as descending fibres from the frontal eye fields. Cortico-bulbar fibres – the motor supply to the head – travel in the genu. The posterior limb contains descending corticospinal fibres, as well as ascending thalamocortical projections to the sensory cortex. The blood supply of the internal capsule is through the anterior circulation, with supply from the anterior and middle cerebral arteries, and anterior choroidal arteries.

13. The thalamus.

A. Is separated from the lentiform nucleus by the posterior limb of the internal capsule.

B. Is connected to the thalamus of the other side by the massa intermedia.

C. Is part of the forebrain.

D. Is separated from the hypothalamus by the hypothalamic sulcus.

E. Is divided into different nuclear masses by the internal medullary lamina.

All true.

The thalamus is a component of the diencephalon, which is part of the forebrain. It is a paired structure, each thalamus lying lateral to the 3rd ventricle, the two being linked through the massa intermedia. The hypothalamic sulcus runs horizontally across the diencephalon separating the thalamus from the hypothalamus. The thalamus lies in close proximity to the basal ganglia, with which it has reciprocal connections. The thalamus is separated from the lentiform nucleus by the posterior limb of the internal capsule. The internal medullary lamina separates the thalamus into functionally different nuclear masses.

14. The ventricular system of the brain.

A. The corpus callosum forms the roof of the lateral ventricles.

B. CSF is produced only in the lateral ventricles.

C. The 3rd ventricle communicates with the 4th ventricle *via* the interventricular foramen of Munro.

D. The cerebral aqueduct runs through the midbrain and pons.

E. The thalamus forms the lateral wall of the 3rd ventricle.

True:	A E
False:	B C D

The lateral ventricles are two cavities lying within the cerebral hemispheres. These cavities are lined with ependyma and filled with CSF. CSF is produced by the choroid plexus found in the lateral, 3rd and 4th ventricles. The lateral ventricles are C-shaped, and made up of a frontal (anterior) horn, body, occipital (posterior) horn and a temporal (inferior) horn. The roof is the corpus callosum. The two anterior horns are separated medially by the septum pellucidum. They communicate with the 3rd ventricle *via* an interventricular foramen.

Behind the interventricular foramen lies the body, and the posterior and inferior horns. The body is bounded medially by the septum pellucidum and fornix, and laterally by the body of the caudate nucleus. The thalamus forms the floor. The posterior horn extends into the occipital lobe, while the inferior horn extends into the temporal lobe. The 3rd ventricle is bounded anteriorly by the lamina terminalis, with the thalamus forming the lateral wall, and the hypothalamus lying inferolaterally. It communicates with the 4th ventricle through the cerebral aqueduct, which runs through the midbrain to open into the 4th ventricle at the ponto-mesencephalic junction. In addition, two lateral apertures (foramina of Lushka) and a median aperture (foramen of Magendie) allow the 4th ventricle to communicate with the subarachnoid space of the cerebellopontine angle and cisterna magna, respectively.

15. The blood supply of the brain.

A. The anterior choroidal artery is a branch of the anterior cerebral artery.

B. The posterior communicating artery is found in the interpeduncular fossa.

C. The basilar artery supplies the brainstem.

D. The ICA terminates lateral to the optic chiasma.

E. The posterior cerebellar artery is a terminal branch of the basilar artery.

F. The pons is supplied by the posterior cerebral artery.

G. Occlusion of the anterior cerebral artery causes weakness in the leg.

H. The middle cerebral artery runs between the frontal and temporal lobes in the lateral sulcus.

I. Broca's area is supplied through branches of the vertebro-basilar system.

J. An occlusion of the anterior cerebral artery may lead to an upper motor neuron weakness.

True:	B C D G H J
False:	A E F I

The blood supply of the brain can be divided into an anterior/carotid circulation and a posterior/basilar circulation. The anterior circulation is derived from the two ICAs. The ICA terminates lateral to the optic chiasma as the anterior and the middle cerebral arteries. The anterior cerebral artery runs in the longitudinal fissure, connected on either side through the anterior communicating artery. It follows the curve of the corpus callosum. It supplies the medial surface of the frontal and parietal lobes. It characteristically supplies the 'leg' area of the motor and sensory cortices. The middle cerebral artery is the largest branch of the ICA. It runs in the lateral fissure between the frontal and temporal lobes, supplying the majority of the brain, including the head and arm areas of the sensory and motor cortices. It also supplies Broca's area. In addition, the ICA gives off the anterior choroidal arteries (supplying the internal capsule and the basal ganglia), ophthalmic arteries and posterior communicating arteries. The latter branch runs into the interpeduncular fossa and connects to the posterior cerebral artery. The posterior circulation is derived from the vertebro-basilar system. The two vertebral arteries unite at the upper margin of the foramen magnum to form the basilar artery. This runs up the basilar pons before terminating as the posterior cerebral artery. Along its course, it gives off branches to the brainstem and cerebellum through the pontine and cerebellar arteries.

Structures contained in, or bounding, the interpeduncular fossa.

A. Olfactory tract.

B. Trochlear nerve.

C. Optic chiasma.

D. Mammillary bodies.

E. Anterior cerebral artery.

True:	C D
False:	A B E

The interpeduncular fossa is a depression in the midbrain that lies between the crura cerebri, with the optic chiasma in front and the pons behind. The roof is formed by the hypothalamus, containing the mammillary bodies and tuber cinerum. The floor is formed by a sheet of arachnoid mater. The oculomotor nerve is contained within the interpeduncular fossa. It emerges from the lateral side to run forward into the lateral wall of the cavernous sinus. The circle of Willis is also closely related to the interpeduncular fossa, with the posterior cerebral artery and posterior communicating artery running into the fossa.

17. **Features of an upper motor neuron lesion.**

A. Increased tendon reflexes.

B. Flaccid paralysis.

C. Positive Babinski sign.

D. Decreased tone.

E. Muscle fasciculations.

True:	A C
False:	B D E

An upper motor neuron lesion is characterised by increased tone with spastic paralysis, increased tendon reflexes, and upgoing plantars – a positive Babinski reflex. This is compared with lower motor neuron lesions which are characterised by decreased tone with flaccid paralysis, muscle wasting and fasciculations, diminished reflexes and downgoing plantars.

18. **The primary motor cortex.**

A. Is found in the postcentral gyrus.

B. Represents an inverted image of the ipsilateral half of the body.

C. Is involved in the planning of movements.

D. Has a blood supply derived from the carotid circulation.

E. Has a blood supply derived from the vertebro-basilar circulation.

True:	D
False:	A B C E

The primary motor cortex is contained in the frontal lobe in the precentral gyrus. It represents an inverted, somatotopic image of the contralateral half of the body. It is involved in the execution of movements. Planning of movements occurs in the premotor cortex. The blood supply is derived from the carotid circulation through the anterior and middle cerebral arteries.

19. The somatosensory cortex.

A. The body is represented somatotopically.

B. The somatosensory cortex is contained in the parietal lobe.

C. Receives afferents from the thalamus.

D. Is damaged in occlusion of the middle cerebral artery.

E. Contains Wernicke's area.

True:	A B C D
False:	E

The somatosensory cortex is contained in the postcentral gyrus of the parietal lobe. Like the motor cortex, the contralateral half of the body is represented in an inverted somatotopic pattern. This area receives afferents from the periphery, which are relayed to it from the thalamus. Blood supply is through the middle and anterior cerebral arteries.

APPENDIX:
ANATOMICAL ABBREVIATIONS

AbPB	Abductor pollicis brevis
ACL	Anterior cruciate ligament
AIVA	Anterior interventricular artery
ASIS	Anterior superior iliac spine
AVN	Atrioventricular node
CC	Common carotid artery
CMC	Carpometacarpal
CSF	Cerebrospinal fluid
DPN	Deep peroneal nerve
EOA	External oblique aponeurosis
EOM	External oblique muscle
FCU	Flexor carpi ulnaris
FDL	Flexor digitorum longus
FDS	Flexor digitorum superficialis
FO	Foramen ovale
FPB	Flexor pollicis brevis
GKT	Guy's, King's and St Thomas's
ICA	Internal carotid arteries
IIA	Internal iliac artery
IJV	Internal jugular vein
IOA	Internal oblique aponeurosis
IOM	Internal oblique muscle
IP	Interphalangeal
IVC	Inferior vena cava
LA	Left atrium
LAD	Left anterior descending artery
LBCT	Left brachiocephalic trunk
LC	Lateral cord
LCA	Left coronary artery
LCCA	Left common carotid artery
LGN	Lateral geniculate nucleus
LIJV	Left internal jugular vein
LMA	Left marginal artery
LSCV	Left subclavian vein
LV	Left ventricle
MAL	Mid-axillary line

MC	Medial cord
MCL	Mid-clavicular line
MCP	Metacarpophalangeal
MCQ	Multiple-choice questions
MRCS	Member of the Royal College of Surgeons
#NOF	Fractured neck of femur
NV	Neurovascular
OP	Opponens pollicis
PA	Pulmonary artery
PC	Posterior cord
PCL	Posterior cruciate ligament
PIP	Proximal interphalangeal
PIVA	Posterior interventricular artery
PSIS	Posterior superior iliac spine
PV	Pulmonary vein
QS	Quadrangular space
RA	Right atrium
RAM	Rectus abdominis muscle
RBCT	Right brachiocephalic trunk
RCA	Right coronary artery
RCCA	Right common carotid artery
RIJV	Right internal jugular vein
RMA	Right marginal artery
RSCV	Right subclavian vein
RTA	Road-traffic-accident
RV	Right ventricle
SAN	Sinoatrial node
SCALP	Skin, Connective tissue, Aponeurosis, Loose connective tissue, and Peritoneum
SI	Small intestine
SIT	Supraspinatus, infraspinatus and teres major
SMA	Superior mesenteric artery
SPN	Superficial peroneal nerve
SVC	Superior vena cava
TAM	Transversus abdominis muscle
TC	Transverse colon
TMJ	Temperomandibular joints
TN	Tibial nerve
TS	Triangular space
TV	Tricuspid valve
VAN	Vein, artery, nerve

INDEX

This book is designed to be a work-book rather than a conventional text book, and as such, it does not have a conventional index.

The layout has been designed to facilitate easy navigation, however, so if you need to locate a specific question, for example to refer to a diagram, use the main **CONTENTS** list on **page v** to find the region of interest and then the **TOPIC CHECK LIST** for the appropriate section, on which each question has a specific page reference.

NOTES